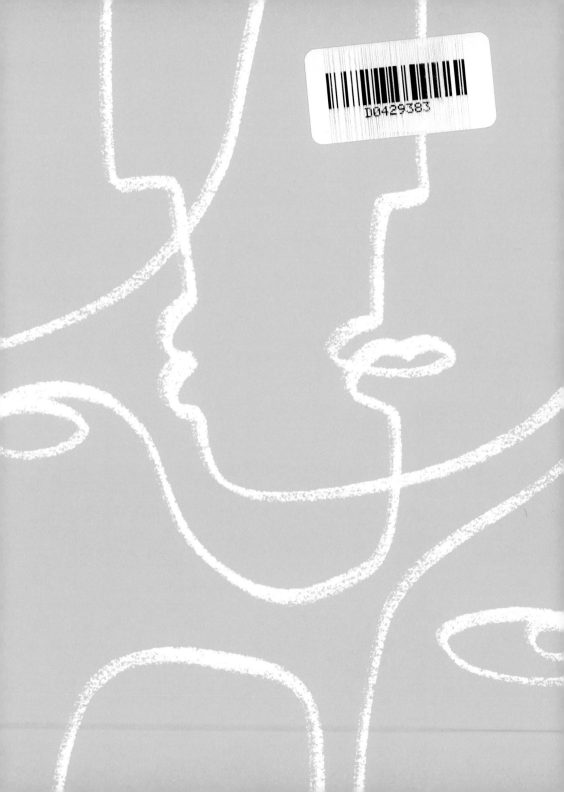

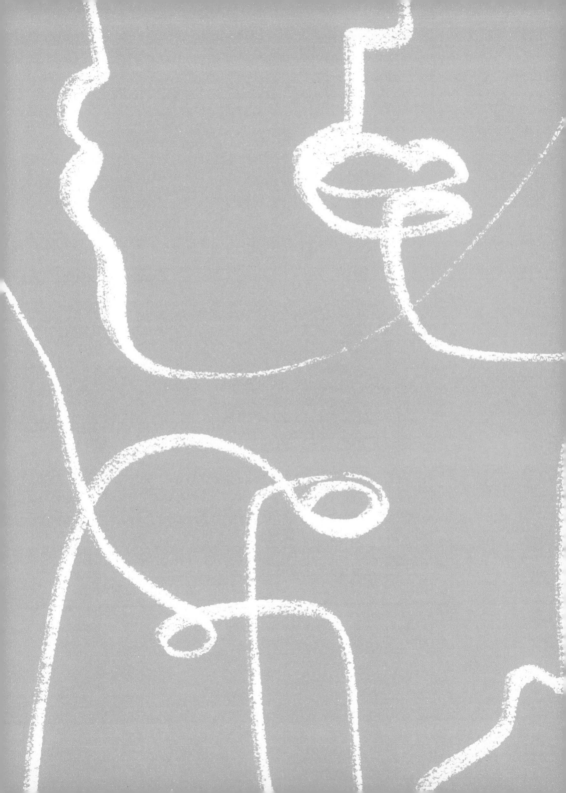

FACE
VALUES

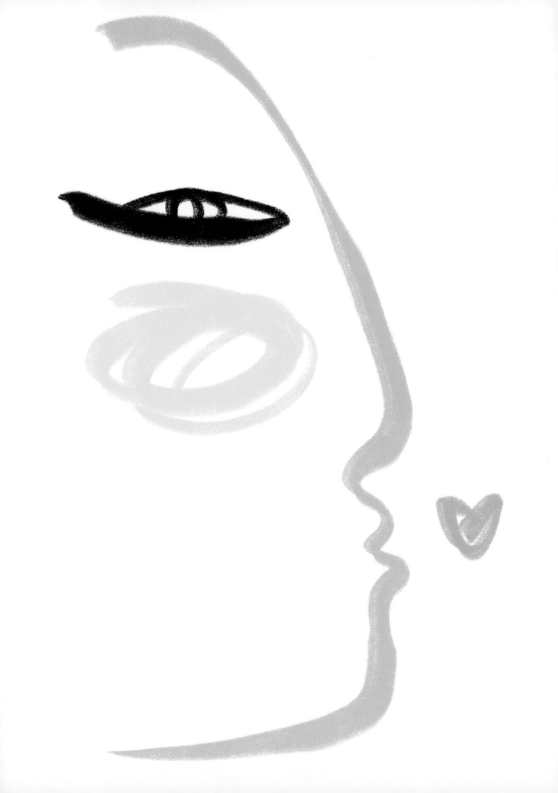

FACE VALUES

Beauty Rituals and Skincare Secrets

Navaz Batliwalla

Contents

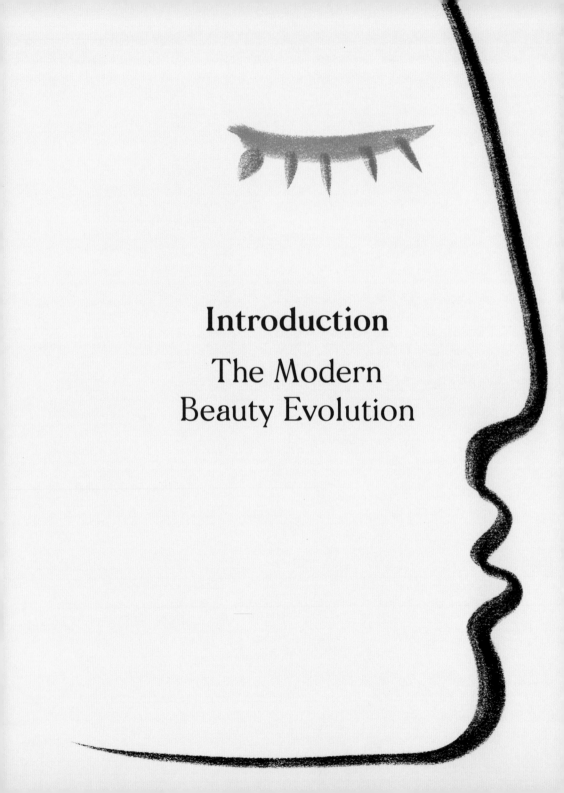

Introduction

The Modern
Beauty Evolution

What is 'beauty' in the 2020s? It feels as though we've been grappling with a similar question since time began, swinging from opulent artifice to the subjective eye of the beholder, to somewhere between the two. My own beauty awakening happened around 2010, reading the voyeuristic pages of the blog Into the Gloss, which catalogued the bathroom-shelf minutiae of the professionally gorgeous. This was accompanied by a chorus of commenters offering their own tips and recommendations, alongside cries of aspirational worship. I lapped up these nuggets, while quickly realizing that talking about 'beauty' is really an excuse to talk about identity: how we see ourselves, and how we want to be seen. When we talk about beauty routines, aren't we really talking about our values, our self-respect and how we feel about our place in society?

For much of the twenty-first century, external beauty has been performative and optimized. Thanks to social media, our own personal *Truman Shows* have portrayed our visages as soulless, filtered avatars. Increasingly, life imitates art with the normalization of Botox and dermal fillers, easily acquired through lunchtime 'tweakments' from the local drugstore or clinic. The rise of the 'Instagram Face' – smooth-browed, plump-cheeked, blemish-free – and accompanying anti-ageing and perfectionist language feels insidiously discriminatory. God forbid one should 'suffer' from fine lines or blemishes!

While the traditional beauty industry continues to push an external beauty agenda that favours the cis-gender male gaze, there has been a counter-shift towards a more achievable beauty ideal driven by fourth-wave feminism and the gender-fluid movement. This is reinforced by the new generation of start-up brands that promote a more positive message of self-acceptance and inclusivity. There's a focus on looking 'well' and an empowered interest in the science of skin health. Brands such as Hiki (deodorant), Glossier (skincare) and Oui the People (shaving and bodycare) have reframed the narrative of sweat, pores and body hair, reminding us that 'flawless' is an advertising construct, not a reality.

Although history has conspired to serve us unobtainable ideals, the twentieth and twenty-first centuries also brought their fair share of beauty influencers: the artists, tastemakers and accidental activists who represent a positive, non-standard

'Although history has conspired to serve us unobtainable ideals, the twentieth and twenty-first centuries also brought their fair share of beauty influencers: the artists, tastemakers and accidental activists who represent a positive, non-standard way to show up.'

Opposite, clockwise from top left: Artist Georgia O'Keeffe at Ghost Ranch, New Mexico, 1964; Mexican painter Frida Kahlo expressed beauty on her own terms; *Nude Maria Combing Her Hair* by Cassi Namoda conveys the everyday rituals of self-care.

way to show up. The handsome, monastic appearance of the painter Georgia O'Keeffe (1887–1986) is all of a sudden relevant, coupled with her appetite for organic eating, using ingredients foraged from the land surrounding her famous Ghost Ranch in New Mexico. The emotional art of Frida Kahlo (1907–1954) expressed the trauma of a near-fatal pelvic and spinal injury, while outwardly she used make-up and perfume as tools to construct her striking persona. A century on, millennial fans would pay homage to her unapologetically unplucked brows. Cindy Sherman, poster girl for questioning identity through art, makes us confront our own humanity through her camera lens, while Elizabeth Peyton's tender portraits of 1990s music idols have helped to turn the tables on toxic masculinity.

From a style perspective, I'm forever inspired by the androgyny of Tina Chow (1950–1992), Patti Smith and Tilda Swinton, and the confidence with which they upend society's hyper-feminine ideals. By the same token, male artists from David Bowie (1947–2016) to Jean-Michel Basquiat (1960–1988) have demonstrated an equally radical pride in being true to their identities.

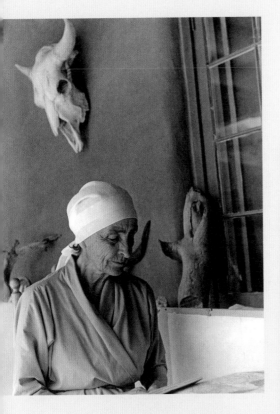

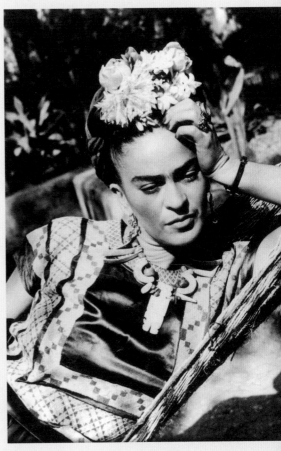

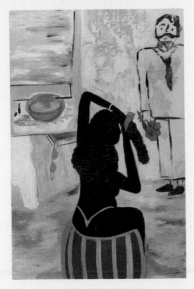

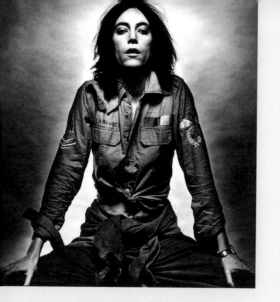

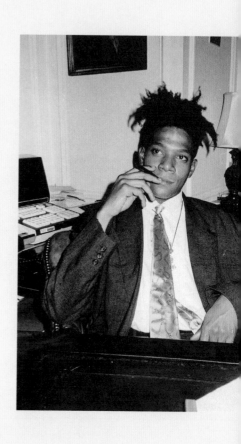

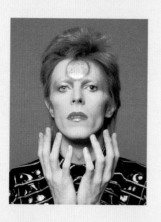

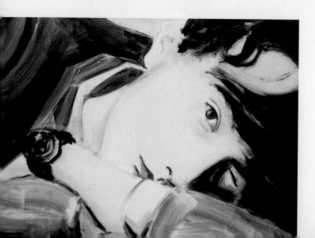

'But let's be clear. Beauty today isn't limited to how we look. Internal beauty – how we feel – has taken centre stage during recent turbulent times.'

Opposite, clockwise from top left: 'Punk poet' Patti Smith has been a trailblazer for anti-perfectionists. Painter Jean-Michel Basquiat's nonchalant look was as uncompromising as his art; *Jarvis* encapsulates Elizabeth Peyton's portrayal of masculinity; the chameleon-like identities of David Bowie inspired a generation of fashion lovers.

For decades beauty has equalled youth, but the pioneers overthrowing that notion continue to do their work. Isabella Rossellini, Bethann Hardison and Lauren Hutton have modelled well into their sixties and seventies, encouraged by a new generation of consumers who welcome anti-ageism. And on the Internet, the ardent followers of Linda V. Wright and That's Not My Age blogger Alyson Walsh prove that there's plenty of purchase power in the silver pound.

But let's be clear. Beauty today isn't limited to how we look. Internal beauty – how we feel – has taken centre stage during recent turbulent times. The concept of self-care dates back to ancient Greece, when Socrates referred to the 'care of the self' as care of the soul. More recently, 1960s feminists used self-care as a means to teach women about female health, long before the term was hijacked by the corporate wellness brigade pushing luxury vitamin water packaged for 'the gram'.

This century's self-care rituals needn't cost money, but they may cost a little time. And so they should. There are proven benefits to taking time for a magnesium bath, facial massage or sensorial oil cleanse. This is the anti-optimized part of beauty, dedicated to maintaining equilibrium or resetting the system.

Just ask the Japanese, the Chinese and the Indians, who are firm believers in mindful rituals and routines. Despite the 'perfectionist presentation' we see on social media, it's OK if your face cloths aren't pristine or your bathroom tiles are chipped. You don't have to perform your ritual on social; in fact, it's far better to make the bathroom a no-phone zone.

While we're not immune to the lure of tactile packaging and chic branding, there's evidence that the hyper-consumerist element of beauty and self-care is subsiding. In 2019 the consumer insight company Mintel reported that 28 per cent of women in the UK had reduced the number of products in their skincare routines, mirroring a preference for products containing fewer, purer ingredients. This also tallies with the zero-waste movement. Single-use plastic bottles, razors and even lipstick

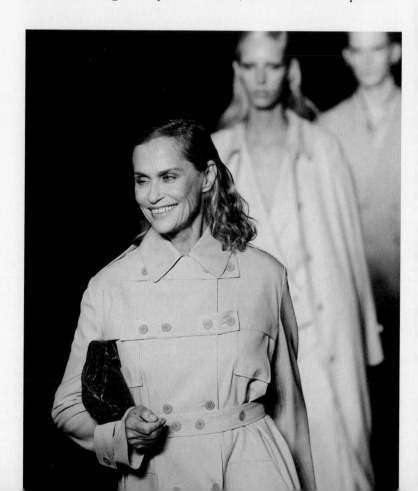

Right: Fashion advocate and sometime model Bethann Hardison champions representation in front of the camera and behind the scenes.

Opposite: Lauren Hutton and Bottega Veneta endorse anti-ageism on the spring/summer 2017 runway.

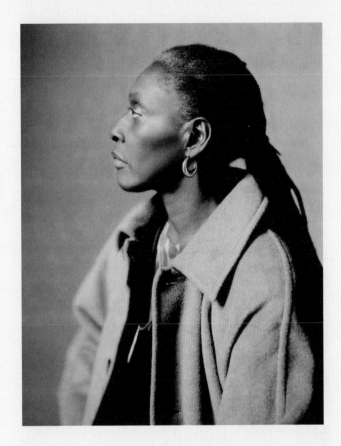

cases are being swapped for beautiful glass containers and refill services that preserve the planet's resources.

In the following pages we'll explore some of these resetting rituals and the new guard of beauty advocates who embody their benefits. Some of the individuals steering this quiet revolution have been on my radar for a long time; others were recommended to me; and others still found their way into my orbit fortuitously. Despite being very different, all are doing their thing to spread a positive message of self-acceptance, one that proves the power of beauty today is much more than skin deep.

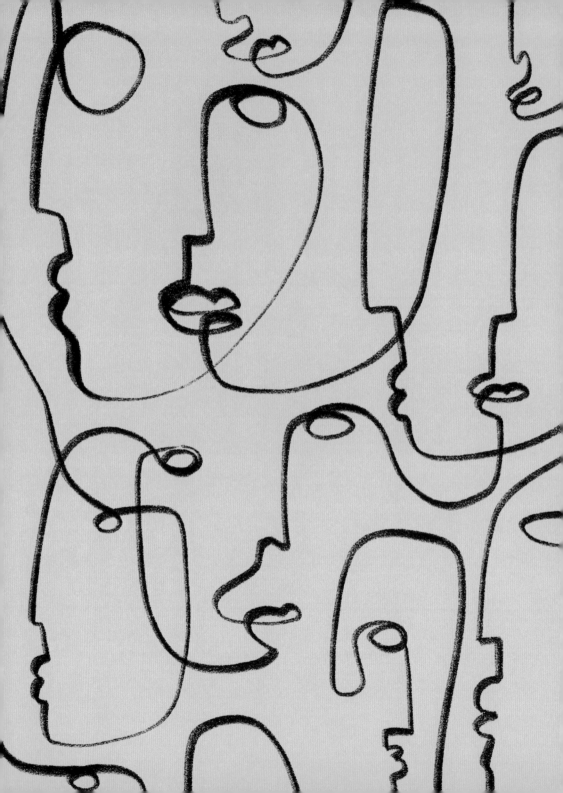

The Ritualists

Inviting us into their private sanctuaries,
the ritualists talk through their beauty
philosophies, influences and personal practices
that get them through the day. From an anti-
perfectionist Brazilian footwear designer to
a Japanese massage therapist, they offer us
their secrets to looking and feeling good.

Theresa Williams

CO-FOUNDER OF
CELSIOUS ECO-LAUNDRETTE

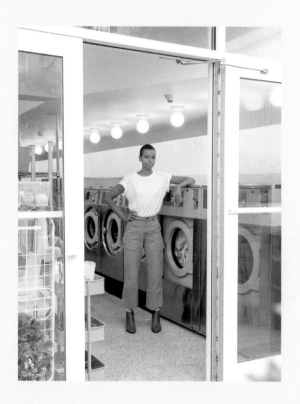

For Theresa Williams, co-owner of New York's
first eco-conscious laundrette, Celsious, a minimalist
approach to beauty comes naturally. She grew up
in Bavaria, where her hippie mother influenced her
fuss-free aesthetic, while the time and money constraints
of entrepreneurial life inform her signature cropped hair.
For this former product designer, simple pleasures come
from storing home-made face oils in Murano glass bottles.

My sister Corinna was working as a fashion journalist and moved to New York for a job. We grew up in Germany, where most people have a washing machine in their house, and when she moved to New York and used a laundromat for the first time, she wasn't happy with the experience. So she decided to create her own, and roped me in by asking me to help with the interior design. Celsious opened in 2018.

My beauty journey was strongly influenced by my upbringing. Our mother is German and we always used very natural products at home. She was pretty strict about not letting my sister and me wear make-up at the age our classmates were experimenting with it. She was more of an eco-conscious hippie, so I think she wasn't comfortable with us at 12 or 13 wearing make-up, and she didn't want us to use products with unnecessary chemicals in them. I was definitely bummed out at the time, but now I do respect the choice my mother made.

I was fortunate to have pretty good skin. I had eczema, but I never had breakouts. Generally, everything I do in terms of skincare has always revolved around finding products that will be good for my skin. Certain things give me rashes – anything with synthetic fragrances, synthetic ingredients, even essential oils. My main goal is making sure my skin is healthy, that's what's driven me for the last 20 years in terms of taking care of my body.

Growing up in Bavaria, there weren't many people who looked like us. There were no hairdressers who could deal with our curly hair, and our mother, being white, also didn't really know what to do with it. We probably would've preferred to fit in a bit more, but we had to find our own path.

I never straightened my hair. Strong chemicals were a big no-no, but I definitely tried to braid my hair down so that it looked more like longer hair. Then I ended up having dreadlocks for six or seven years, so my hair grew really long. I loved the style; I was also a little bit of a hippie back then. But it was also so I didn't have to go anywhere to get my hair cut, because nobody could do it, so that was self-maintaining and self-sustaining. Then, when I wanted something a little less heavy and bulky, really my only option was to shave my hair off, because I couldn't undo the dreadlocks or anything. That's when I realized short hair really suits me. So for the last ten years I've shaved my own hair.

Minimalism is a great time- and money-saver. That's something that can be a little hard to talk about when starting your own business. When you're running a business, you put everything you have into it, and you initially don't have a ton of money. So being frugal with the resources I do have is something that's still driving some of my choices.

Dr Bronner's Castile bar soap is all I use in the shower. I try to be as low-waste as possible, so I like a bar of soap that's just wrapped in a piece of paper. It's mild enough for me to use on my hair-slash-scalp and for the rest of my body. So that's basically all I have in the shower.

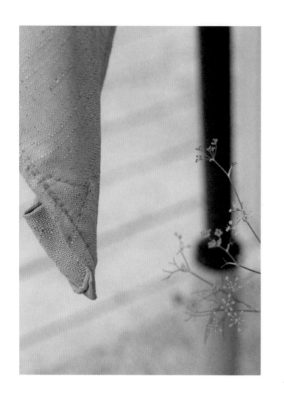

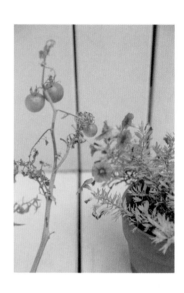

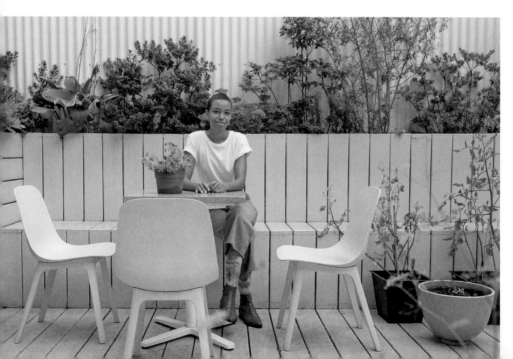

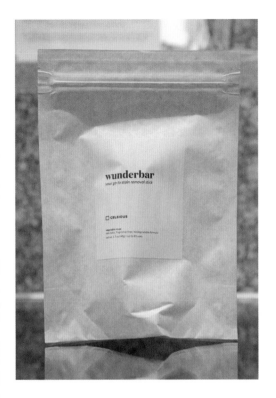

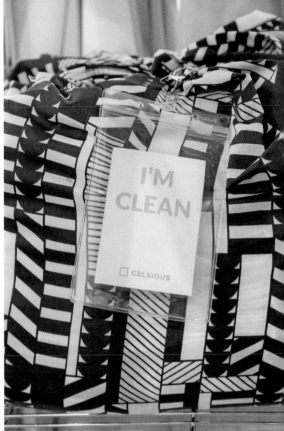

In the mornings and evenings I rinse my face with warm water and massage in a castor-oil blend that I mix myself. I just researched it online. Whenever I had flare-ups, I looked for oils that might help with that and experimented. Because I don't wear make-up, there's nothing much to take off, other than rinsing away the New York City grime at the end of the day. I use the oil as an oil cleanser, but I kind of leave it on.

One of our clients is a holistic massage studio, and I learned how to use the Gua Sha massage stone from the owner. So if I don't have time for anything else, I brush my teeth and massage my face for a few minutes morning and night. Those are my non-negotiables.

I've never been a beauty product junkie. The few speciality products I use tend to be made by people I know personally. Runako is a brand owned by friends of ours who just launched a really great body butter with organic ingredients. When it comes to supporting a small business, I think that's money well spent. We also sell Runako in our space.

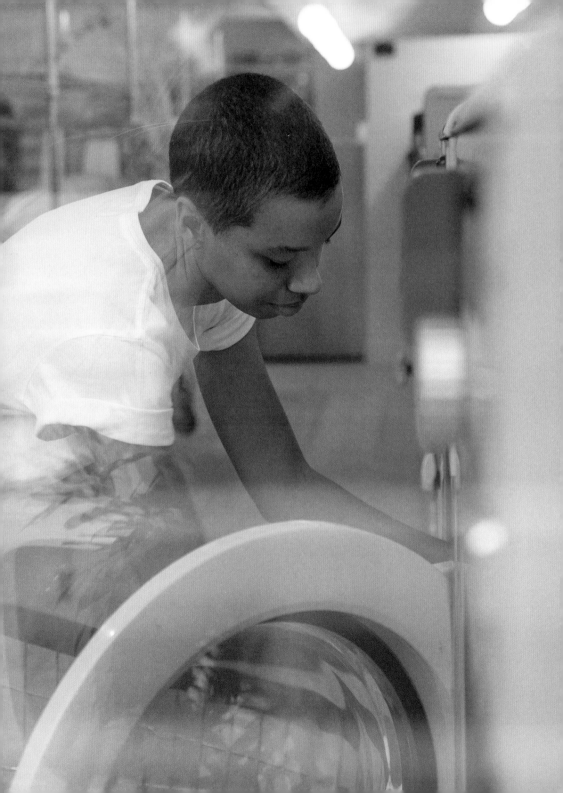

I admit I don't have all the work-life strategies figured out. It's always top of my list to find a healthier balance, but I think that's the case for everyone. I'm naturally a perfectionist and a person who overthinks and over-worries, but I've come to a point where I can control a lot of those feelings, so that helps.

The biggest issue is being able to quiet my mind, so meditation is still something I dabble in. I find it incredibly hard to not think about my to-do list. That's why I like yoga, because I'm focused on something else – on movement, or, if I'm doing hot yoga, on the sensation of being slightly uncomfortable. It's pretty much the only way I can keep myself from thinking about work.

In our bathroom we have mirrored cabinets, which I love, because there's no clutter. Not having my bathroom cabinet full of products I use only occasionally is very important to me. There are a couple of shelves where I keep my things, and I try to organize them every couple of weeks. My husband has more than me, and he likes to experiment with products. He's always on the lookout for something for his beard and something for his hair.

For my facial oil, which is my main face product, I got a really beautiful Murano glass bottle. When you make your own products, you usually end up putting them in empty kombucha bottles or Mason jars. But I thought for a product I use every day, it would be nice to have something that feels a little more luxurious. So I have this nice bottle in different colours with a glass stopper. Using that twice a day brings me a lot of joy.

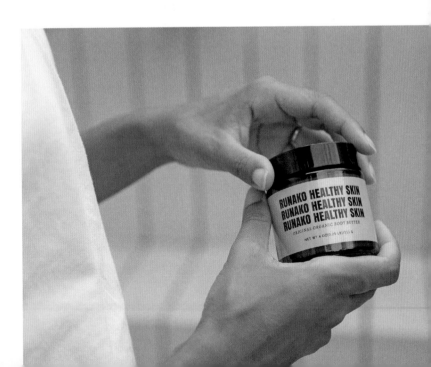

Ruth Barry

BAKER AND OWNER OF
BLACK ISLE BAKERY

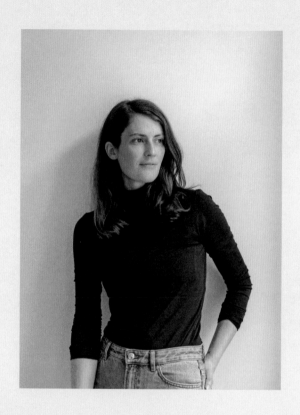

Growing up in Scotland, Ruth Barry was the girl
who loved make-up and performing. After studying
at Edinburgh College of Art and getting a taste of the
New York and London art scenes, she became disillusioned by
the commercial reality of the art world, which led her to an
apprenticeship with the Parisian bakery Du Pain et des Idées.
She is now settled in Berlin, where the Black Isle Bakery
is her stage, and dog walking and massage her therapy.

I grew up on the Black Isle in the highlands of Scotland. I was into style and how I looked from a really early age. My mum was very anti all that stuff, which I think just encouraged me.

When I was very young I started highland dancing. That was very rigid, when what I really wanted was to be a ballerina, because they got to have cool outfits and nice make-up and hairdos. And then I discovered disco dancing. I was very stagey. Because my parents didn't think performing was a serious career path, I was really drawn to this performative expression.

I studied sculpture at Edinburgh College of Art and graduated in 2008, assuming that I would be an artist. After an internship at the Guggenheim in New York, I moved to London and worked for Counter Editions, which made limited-edition artworks with some of the world's most famous artists. It was incredible, but being part of the art world destroyed the illusion that there was something special about art. I had to find a way to make things and be comfortable with the commerce that would surround that.

Baking was my therapy. There's something very nourishing about making a product that you then share with other people. I had also spent my early twenties fighting eating disorders. I started to get help with that and feel better about my body and about myself. It became even more important to be making things that were delicious and that I could share with other people.

I reached out to Christophe Vasseur at Du Pain et des Idées, and he offered me an opportunity to do an apprenticeship with him. Later, I set up the Black Isle Bakery and decided to move to Berlin, because I was dating someone who lived here and also because I wanted to live somewhere that wasn't prohibitively expensive.

I started out supplying other cafes in the city, but my goal was always to have a shop. I found a space and started renovations. Then we discovered by accident that it wasn't legally a commercial space. It took me another year to find the space that I ended up with.

Every business person I know has had a major business struggle of some description. It definitely sorts people into those who are made to do what they're doing and those who are not. I have a little dog, and I think in some ways that's what got me through. No matter what was going on in my life, I had to take her out, even if only for 15 minutes. Those walks helped me to take some deep breaths and get over what I was going through.

When I finish work I'm exhausted. It's constant physical effort, and my brain is constantly engaged. But it's the stage I've found where I don't have to be at the front with the glitter and the red lipstick and earrings, but I can show my style and creativity in a completely different way. I take it so seriously because every little piece of the performance has to be right.

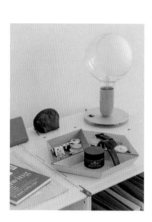

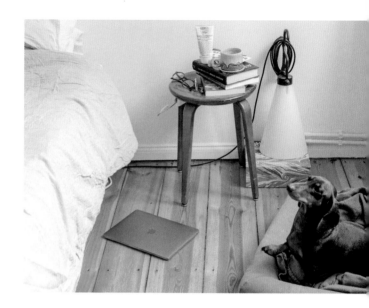

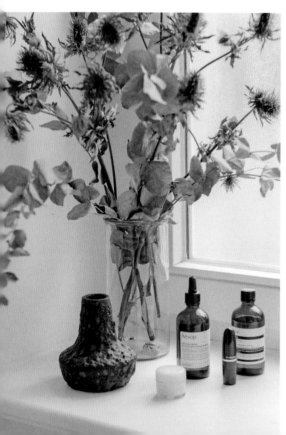

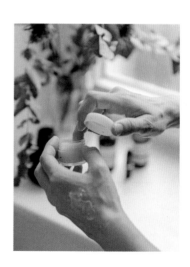

I don't actually cleanse my skin, I just wash it with water. I have moisturizers and eye creams and very simple make-up and that's it. I'm lucky that my wake-up call is only 5 am. I brush my teeth, put on eye cream, moisturizer, a little bit of concealer under my eyes, some gel through my eyebrows and some blush and I'm ready to go.

If I'm going out I wear red lipstick, and that's about it. If you find the perfect red lipstick you really don't need much more if it's applied properly. Maybe I would wear a little bit of mascara, but usually I keep it simple. I used to love red lipstick when I had short hair, because short hair is so androgynous. When I wanted to feel more feminine, then it was a big *pow*, there it is!

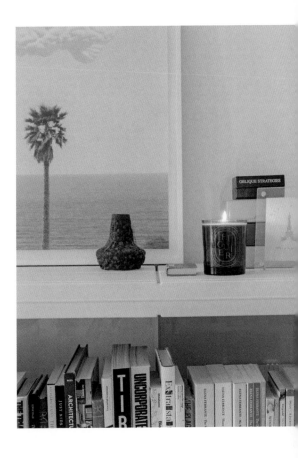

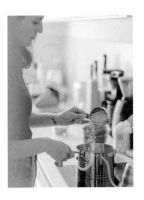

A friend set up a reformer Pilates studio. It makes you feel strong after one session, and that's amazing. I also downloaded this really good app called GLO. It's $15 a month and they have tons of online tutorials for yoga, Pilates, meditation. If I can't make it to the studio, I can do that at home.

The massage therapist Ryoko Hori is one of those people who has magic fingers. I get a full-body massage working on pressure points; there is something very meditative about seeing her. Her treatment rooms are very, very simple, with beautiful little glass bottles of magic potions everywhere. She herself has this amazing calming presence. It's an opportunity to have somebody touch your body in a way that encourages you to let go.

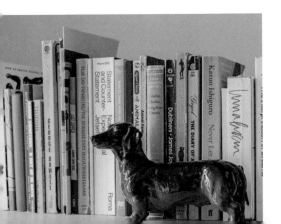

Thakoon Panichgul

FASHION DESIGNER AND FOUNDER
OF *HOMMEGIRLS*

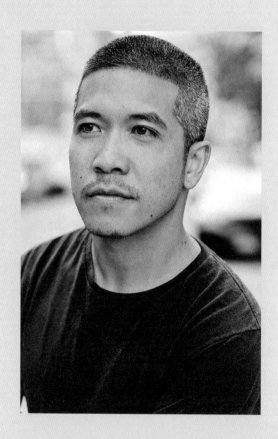

Fashion designer and founder of *HommeGirls* magazine,
Thakoon Panichgul celebrates the anti-male gaze
of his female muses.

I grew up not really fussy about beauty. For me it's more about keeping clean than being finicky about skincare. That said, being Asian, with an Asian mom who is more regimented than ever about her skin, I'm constantly being reminded to wear daily sunscreen, even on my arms, and even on hazy or cloudy days.

My motto is to moisturize! I was never really into anything more than cleanser and moisturizer. But now that I'm in my forties, I'm definitely paying more attention to things like vitamin E and C creams and CBD oils. I use Jason brand vitamin E cream and vitamin C oil for the skin. It's a simple drugstore brand. When you're out in the sun and water, the cream is nice to help your skin heal while moisturizing. I use Superflower CBD moisturizer as well as Saint Jane CBD oil. Both are good because they help to even out the skin tone and give you a fresh look.

I got into scents about five years ago. I used to be so allergic, but for some reason now the right scents are great. I wear Comme des Garçons' Wonderoud, Frédéric Malle's Monsieur., Nasomatto's Duro and some Italian pharmacy brands. Sometimes I'll layer an oil note on top of the scent, just to dirty it up. I'm drawn to wood- and tobacco-based scents.

Working in fashion, you learn a lot about how rules of style are created and fabricated. The women I love are the ones who don't care that much about what others think of them; it makes their style much more interesting. It's a philosophy that culminated in what *HommeGirls* (my magazine for women who love menswear) is all about. When women dress for themselves, they start to discover their personal style: the way a shirt hangs, the way a jacket drapes. It turns into proportion play with simple pieces that are classic and timeless. That's the *HommeGirls* spirit.

I grew up in Thailand, in a culture where women like to wear make-up and dress up a lot, because that's what they're taught. But I don't believe in that approach fully because I think it's more to do with the male gaze than for yourself. I think in today's times, rules are being broken and ideas of how women look are more complex. They should be, because everyone is different.

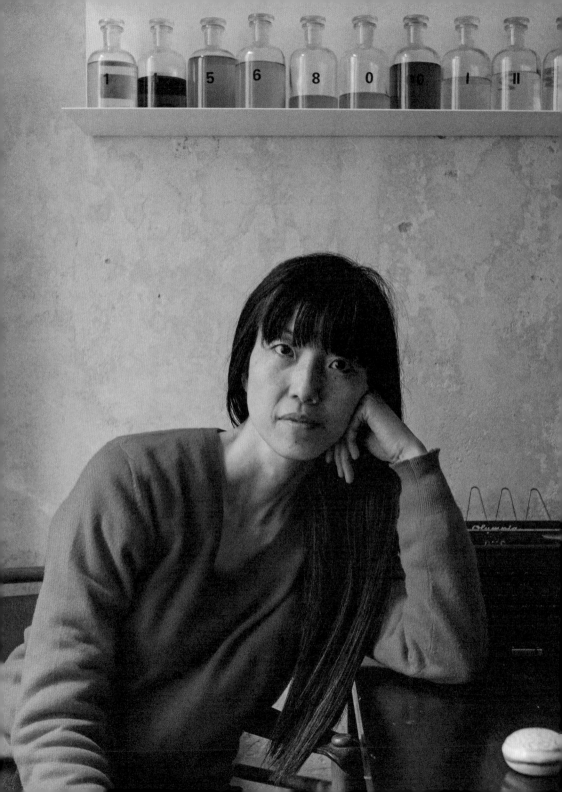

Ryoko Hori

MASSAGE THERAPIST

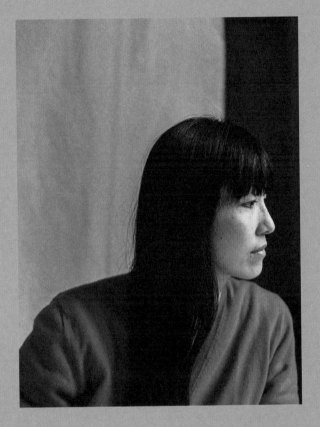

Born in Osaka, Ryoko Hori studied fashion in Tokyo, went on to work for a Japanese fashion designer after spending time in France, then moved to Australia and India to learn about Ayurveda and different societies. She is now based in Berlin, where her space, Senses Salon, helps clients overcome visual overload with massage treatments and aromatherapy. Her secret to wellbeing involves too much tea and taking 'just ten minutes' to sit.

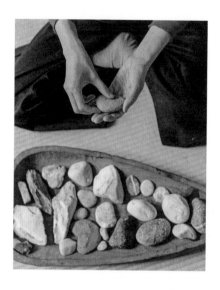

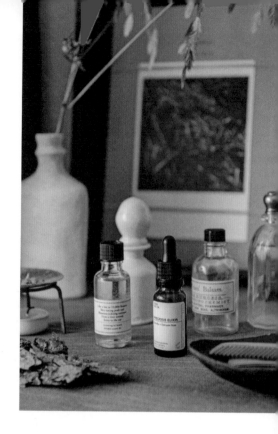

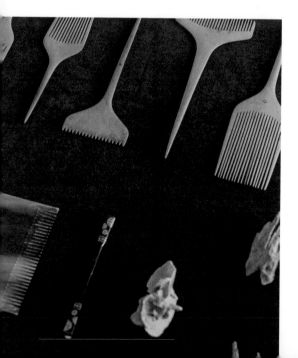

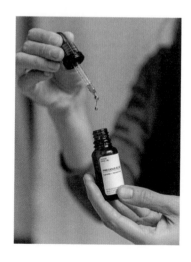

I've enjoyed using my hands since childhood.
My grandmum taught me how to knit, how to sew
and how to make things with my hands. Somehow
I started making clothes for myself, and at 18 I went
to Tokyo to study fashion design. I went to Paris for
three years, then worked in Tokyo for Issey Miyake,
which was inspiring. But the Japanese work ethic
is very intense, and I became very interested in the
connection between mind and body. Once I had
thought about my life and what I wanted to do,
I decided to do something for myself.

I'm very much a visual person, but right now the
visual is dominating the other senses. We don't use
our sense of smell enough; when we eat, we decide
before tasting based on what we see. I want to move
away from visual overload. It's interesting how you
process information without seeing.

Scent is intuitive. It's connected to memory and
emotion, and it affects our mental and physical
condition. At Senses Salon, which I run with my
partner, Daniel, we want to focus on the senses
that are 'lost'. There's nowhere you can go to smell,
apart from perfume shops! Maybe to the garden, but
we want to create somewhere that gives people an
opportunity to smell without buying things. These
days 'perfume' is thought of as an artificial, alcohol-
based liquid, but we have natural wood in which
the perfume comes from the smoke. And we have
different types of material to smell for pleasure,
or for medicinal or ceremonial reasons.

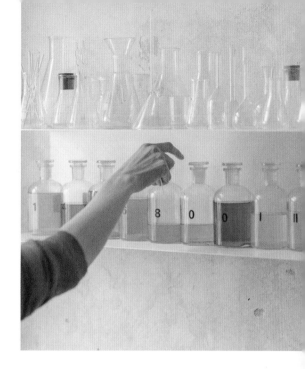

We collect incense boxes from Japan; they're
very special because you can't find them easily. It's
a tradition that's slowly disappearing. I also like
Japanese antiques and collecting stones when we go
somewhere. We use them for the bath.

**Traditionally, the Japanese had a more holistic way
of seeing the body.** But even in Japan now, because
of mass media, the modern approach is about trying
to put creams on the skin without thinking about
why certain conditions happen. I think if you have
lots of product, it can make skin complaints worse.
People are overloading their skin with product.

To me it's not a bad thing to have wrinkles.
I actually think it's very sweet and cute, so I don't
understand the appeal of Botox and fillers. Also,
it's never-ending. It's very much the image you get
from mass media; it's like being brainwashed.

At our salon, we offer different experiences –
massage, treatments – and we host workshops. We're
very connected to the things we have in our shop. We
have the artists and the makers; we wanted to show
things that are handmade from organic materials.

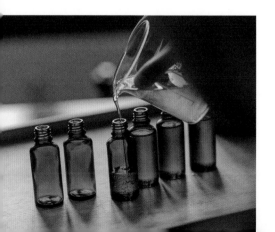

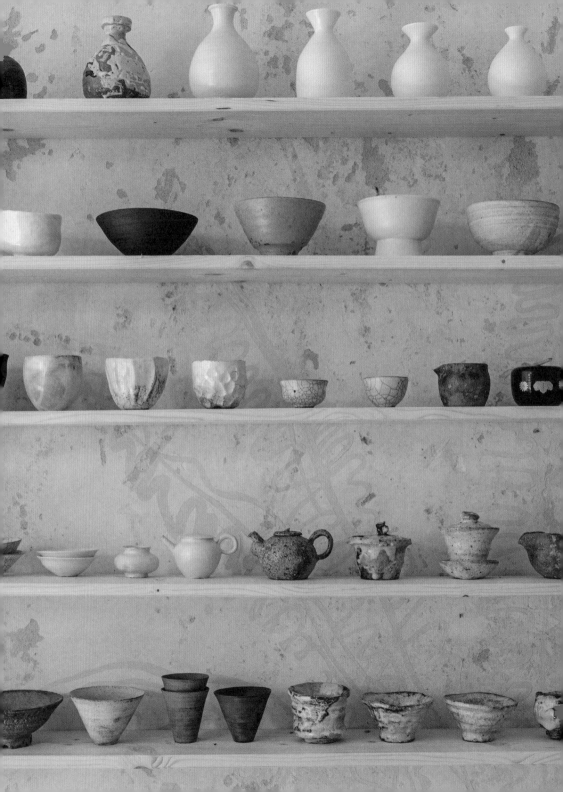

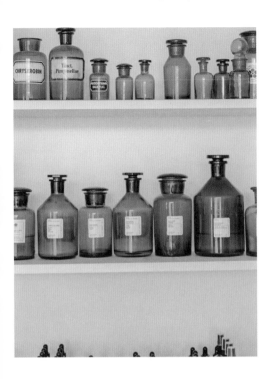

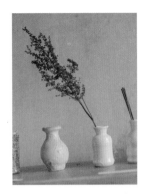

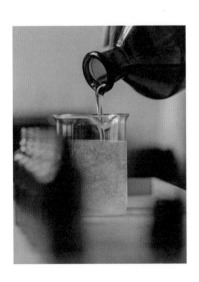

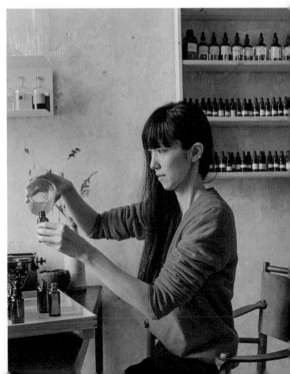

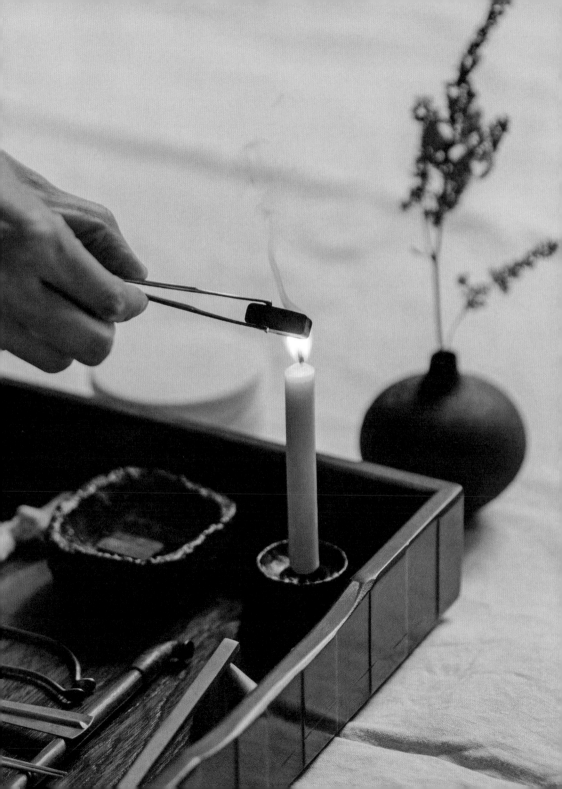

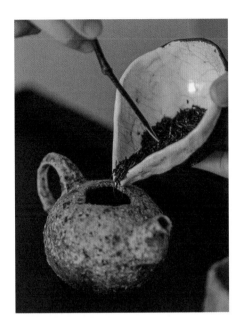

My favourite beauty spot in Berlin is a very beautiful private collection museum called the Feuerle Collection. You can only visit by guided tour, and it's so inspiring. It's a collection of contemporary art as well as antique furniture from fifteenth-century China. Before going into the exhibition you wait in a dark room and listen to music, so it's a very meditative, sensory space.

Here in Berlin, people take time. Although rents have become more expensive and people have to work harder to afford them, it's still very like a village. We have lots of parks. Sometimes you go out for a drink in the middle of the week and lots of people hang out in the park. In Tokyo, no way, people are always working. Rent is expensive in Berlin, but there's still a sense of freedom here.

Most of my time is in the treatment room, so that's where I listen to music. Nils Frahm is a big inspiration. He has lots of styles, but the one I like is very pure, sometimes just one sound. When I work on the human body, I go very deep, so that's very interesting to listen to.

My tsubaki face oil combines rose, tsubaki and rosehip oils. It's a calming and anti-inflammatory elixir, which you apply by patting it on to the face. Rose is antibacterial and good for acne. Tsubaki is a very interesting Japanese ingredient that comes from the camellia flower. In Sumo sport, the hair is often treated with tsubaki oil, which is good for the hair and skin. It doesn't get greasy on the skin surface, and it helps elasticity. It's perfect for everything.

I'm not a morning person. I don't eat, I don't wake up early. I drink tea very slowly – my guilty pleasure is drinking lots of Japanese black tea. It should be taken in moderation, but sometimes I have too much and my nervous system can't cope!

I try to meditate once a day, but even if I don't have time I'll take ten minutes just to sit down. You can do different things, but it's very important sometimes to sit down and do nothing.

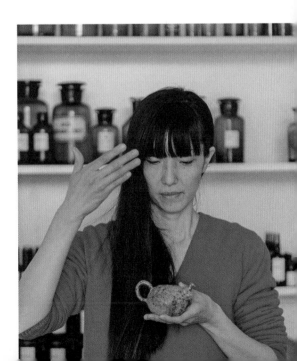

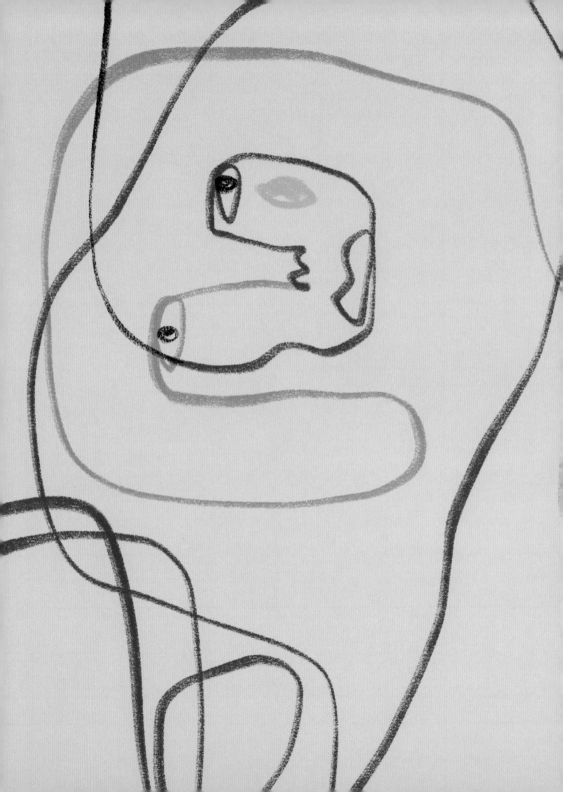

The Rituals:
Self-care and Wellness

Think of self-care and most people conjure twee images of cashmere eye masks and Pinterest slogans. Yet the origin is much more noble. The idea of self-care emerged in the late 1960s as a means for radical feminists and members of the Black Panther Party in the United States to educate and assist marginalized communities ignored by the medical establishment.

Today, self-care and its close ally, wellness, are tools for us to combat the stress and strife of daily life. Since the introduction of the smartphone, we've become used to constant mental stimulation. If you can't go for a short walk without being plugged into music, a podcast or a messaging app, consider yourself afflicted. But it's not entirely your fault. Social media apps have been cunningly designed to mimic slot machines in order to keep you welded to them. And the smooth, tactile feeling of the device in the palm of your hand? That's what makes the whole experience so damn seductive. It's all a ploy to create a sense of intimacy that you just can't resist.

But we've clearly reached a tipping point. We're so overwhelmed by the tsunami of information, the always-on tech tyranny of the modern workplace and the sheer effort of keeping it all together that Harvard Business School now teaches mental wellness and meditation as part of its management courses. Get ready, then, for an influx of products and services promising to cure every ailment your unstoppable lifestyle can throw at you. In 2020 the wellness industry was worth $4.5 trillion, according to the Global Wellness Summit. It grew twice as fast as the global economy, proof that get-well-quick programmes have become the new get-rich-quick schemes. Don't be surprised to see ads for designer vitamin supplements popping up regularly between influencer endorsements for eco-water bottles and athleisure on your social feeds.

But wellness doesn't have to be an elitist pursuit. 'People are searching for meaning, connection and joy in the simple things because there's so much going on, such an overload of information and movement that it's easy to get spun out,' says Ariana Mouyiaris, founder of Cosmic Cosmic, a ritual and healing space opening in London in 2022, which will offer feel-good activities from meditation to life drawing. Having co-founded a successful beauty brand, MAKE, she left the company in 2019 wanting to create something that felt like a retreat but in an urban environment, where clients could learn, release and heal. An 'existential search' following family trauma brought her to study a variety of holistic practices, eventually combining traditional Eastern therapies with a modern approach.

What these ancient healing therapies have in common is the idea of balancing and resetting our systems. For energy-field-based therapies such as Japanese reiki, Chinese qigong (pronounced 'chee-gun') and Tibetan sound-gong meditation, the aim is to increase general wellbeing by relaxing the mind and body, easing mental and thus physical stress and tension. While they may sound intangible, their benefits are rooted in science.

Put simply, stress triggers inflammation in the body, which over the long term contributes to disease and chronic physical ailments. Recent studies show that mindful meditation training reduces the activity of the genes related to inflammation. Stress is also a key trigger for skin complaints, including acne, psoriasis and eczema. Too much of the stress hormone cortisol causes the skin's natural sebum to thicken, blocking pores and causing acne outbreaks and skin flare-ups.

While the super-dedicated might commit to lengthy yoga or meditation practice and ten-day silent retreats, there are plenty of more accessible ways to cultivate a mindful existence. Try baking bread or scrapbooking, for example, or even kitchen-table pottery. As the British potter Bernard Leach once observed, 'potting is one of the few activities today in which a person can use his natural faculties of head, heart, and hand in balance.'

Then there are micro-meditations, small everyday moments of focus and self-reflection. Or, simply, *consciously* untethering yourself from your tech device. For the Japanese model and translator Taira, it's all about the ritual of making matcha green tea instead of coffee to stay focused during a busy day. They also note the purposeful pace of eating in Japan, chewing slowly (using chopsticks helps), which naturally aids digestion. For Mouyiaris, oral care is the surprisingly enjoyable ritual that gives her the necessary pause. She mentions specifically the age-old Ayurvedic practice of oil pulling, swishing sesame oil around the mouth to loosen debris and prevent the build-up of plaque: 'You can do it for however long it takes you to do the dishes. For me, that's meditation. Whatever you do in your day, just take a moment to be conscious of what you're doing. It's not perfect, but at different points we do the best we can.'

Should time and space permit, head to the great outdoors. Wild swimming in bucolic surroundings and onsen bathing in Japanese hot springs offer physical healing and tranquil contemplation. Florence Nightingale and Charles Darwin were fans of the former, enjoying the endorphin release and immunity boost of the cold plunge. I'm the world's worst swimmer and averse to the cold, so I'd much prefer the latter – a dip in steaming mineral waters wearing nothing but a small towel folded on one's head.

If that all sounds a little too much, even a dog walk or time spent talking to your plants will have mindful benefits. 'I encourage my clients to stop thinking exercise and focus on movement,' says the age-management consultant and nutritionist Karen Cummings-Palmer. 'Being outdoors is the best possible option, soaking up some Vitamin D from the sun, which is essential for bone maintenance as we age, and boosting our circulation.'

Whether active or resting, what matters most is the intention. The Japanese massage therapist and holistic beautician Ryoko Hori tries to meditate once a day, 'but even if I don't have time I'll take ten minutes just to sit down. It's very important to sit down doing nothing. I think it's necessary in this society.' What better excuse to put your feet up and give yourself permission to take a mental-health break?

Isa-Welly Locoh-Donou

REGISTERED NUTRITIONIST
AND WELLNESS COACH

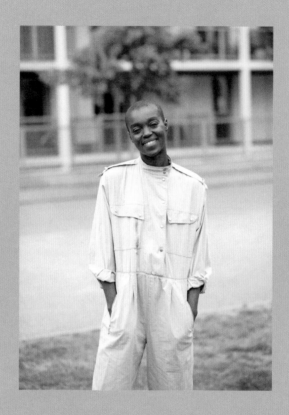

Born and raised in Togo, Isa-Welly Locoh-Donou emigrated
with her family to Paris when she was 12. At 19 she moved
to London to study marketing, but discovered that her real
passion was dance. Following a successful dance career, she
retrained as a nutritionist and now shares her infectious
positivity and energy as a Pilates and wellness coach with a
committed online following.

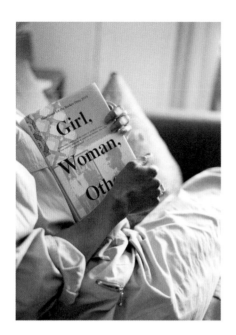

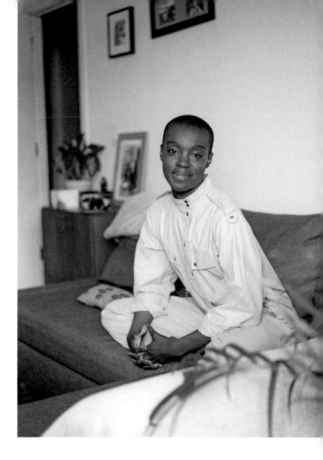

My mum is the most stylish woman ever. She's a pianist and very elegant. And my dad is as well, always suited and booted. At a very young age I was exposed to this elegant but positive attitude – keep your skin as dark as possible, you don't need make-up. I wasn't allowed to wear make-up till I was like 18. My mum doesn't even wear make-up; just powder and that's it.

Clean skin is the big thing for me. And I moisturize a lot. Cleansing oils – that I'll spend time doing. I tend to make a lot of products because I'm big on natural products. I buy the oils in bulk – essential oils, normal oil and fragrance – and I just mix it. I love the end-of-day skincare ritual. It's a routine that says, OK, time to wind down, and it just makes my skin feel better.

I realized I'm a short-hair girl. I tried to grow it and like, hell, no! I cut my hair when I was 20 and I'd just broken up with my first boyfriend. I remember walking on a train in Paris, and I saw this girl. She was shaved and she had these big headphones on and she was just so cool. I thought, oh my God, I need this look. I do a quick shave every week. Fifteen minutes and I'm done.

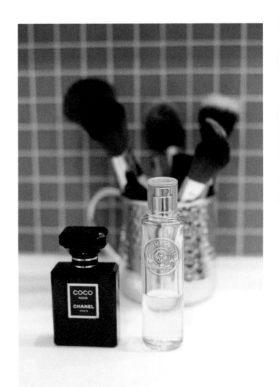

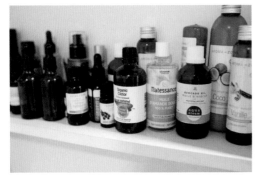

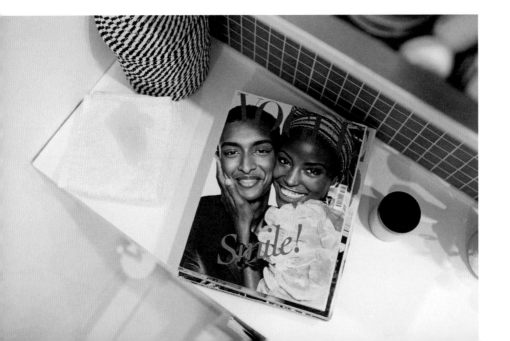

'The emotional wellbeing is really important. Sometimes people eat well and exercise a lot, but they don't feel great. So it's, "OK, what's happening? Why don't you feel good?" I'm not a therapist, but there are times when I have to listen. People just want to talk, to express, and not keep it in.'

I work with people who are at a crossroads, where maybe they had a lifestyle that was a little chaotic and they didn't make space for themselves. That's where I intervene. The emotional wellbeing is really important. Sometimes people eat well and exercise a lot, but they don't feel great. So it's, 'OK, what's happening? Why don't you feel good?' I'm not a therapist, but there are times when I have to listen. People just want to talk, to express, and not keep it in.

I got into Pilates because I injured myself when I was a dancer on tour with Take That in 2007. I always had knee and ankle problems, and it affected my performance. One of my tour managers said I should take up Pilates. I got this incredible teacher who was 75, and I fell in love with it. Then, when I was thinking of retiring, I thought, OK, what can I start doing now to bring in an income? Pilates training took me less than a year, and I started teaching pretty much straight away.

I qualified in Pilates and then I did a wellness coaching qualification. And then I thought, I love learning, but also I don't want to be another influencer who just loves food and giving advice to people online. Studying is hard, but if you have a good why, a big why, you've got a bigger picture and you'll see it through.

'I love learning, but also
I don't want to be another
influencer who just loves food
and giving advice to people
online. Studying is hard, but if
you have a good why, a big why,
you've got a bigger picture and
you'll see it through.'

One of the first things I've learned from building my own brand over the past few years is the importance of preparation. A big key to my success is that I'm so disciplined and rigorous in terms of my time. That's what gives me the freedom to tweak things to make them better, and to do other stuff.

I have a lot of books, because I love reading and I love learning. I have spiritual books, nutrition books and wellness books, and I also love biographies and fiction.

My bathroom's actually quite tidy. I keep it neat because I have a lot of products. Because I make my own oils, I have a lot of prep ingredients, and sometimes I use ten oils to make just one.

I used to have such bad acne. I felt really insecure, especially as I had short hair, because you can't hide. That's when I realized I had to work on it, and that's when I got into wellness and started to understand that what I was eating and my energy, my gut and my moods were affecting my skin.

I like light scents, like Coco Chanel Noir. I like when you smell it when you're close to me. I find that really sexy. But I work a lot one-to-one with people, so I don't want to overpower them with my smell.

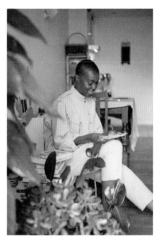
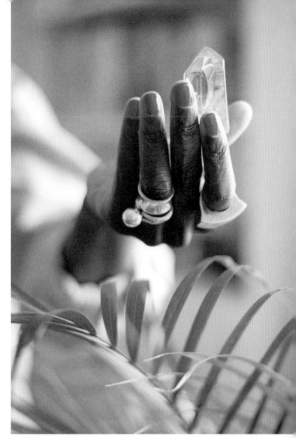
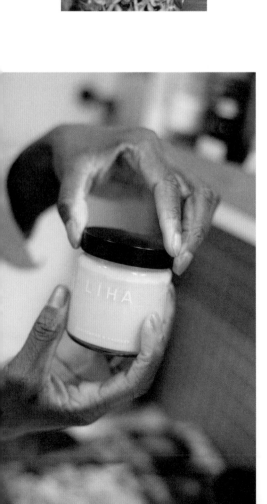
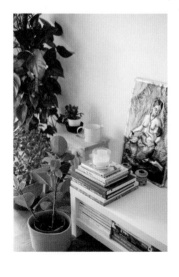

Frédéric Malle

PERFUME PUBLISHER

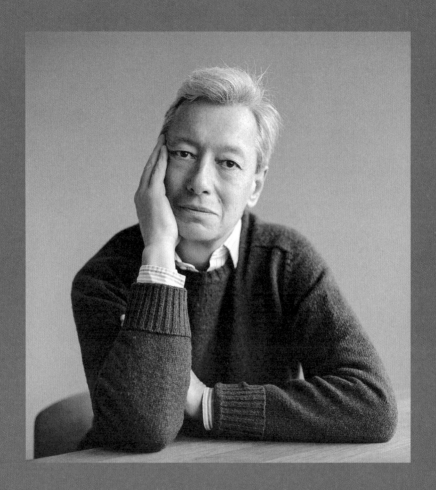

The perfume publisher Frédéric Malle set up his fragrance brand to allow the world's best perfumers to produce unique olfactory works of art under their own names.

My mother, who was not the typical soccer mom, nor the playground type, used to roll our stroller at the Louvre, and my father was one of the best-dressed people I've ever seen. One showed us beauty; the other showed us a kind of understated elegance. This was the basis of my upbringing. Culture, whether it was cinema, music or history, came along.

At the end of the 1990s, luxury perfumery had almost disappeared and the rare person who was attempting to make good perfumes acted as if one could make such products only when referring to the past. I wanted to show the world that perfumery could be another form of contemporary art: modern, luxurious and inventive.

Beauty as a whole is probably what makes me wake up in the morning. I'm a sucker for beauty of any kind – a beautiful person, beautiful music, beautiful architecture. Today I'm wearing Vetiver Extraordinaire, but yesterday I was wearing Geranium pour Monsieur. I use four or five perfumes from our collection, according to my mood.

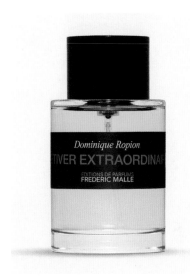

My self-care rituals? I drink Darjeeling tea in the morning, and Lapsang tea in the afternoon. I cried when they had to cover my pool last week [during the Covid-19 pandemic] because I used to swim laps every morning.

I have very simple habits. My routine is limited to our very good Vetiver Extraordinaire Shaving Cream and After Shave, and that's it. Nothing extravagant, I'm old-fashioned that way.

I think great perfumes will always be inventive, specific and very personal. This being said, perfumery relies very much on chemistry to evolve. So as always, novelty in perfumery will be dictated by ingredients. We'll see what the chemists will come up with.

Ariana Mouyiaris

CREATIVE DIRECTOR
AND WELLNESS ENTREPRENEUR

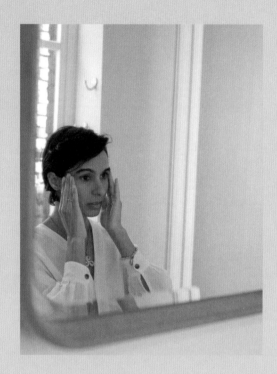

Born in New York to Greek-Cypriot and
American parents, the wellness entrepreneur Ariana
Mouyiaris grew up surrounded by the glamour of the
beauty business. Under the influence of her make-up
manufacturer father, she used her talent as a curator and
creative director to co-found MAKE, an early adopter of
ethically minded beauty practices. Now settled in
East London with her young family, she is focused
solely on her ritual space, Cosmic Cosmic.

I grew up in New York in the 1980s. My father was a chemist who started a beauty manufacturing company by himself, in the late 1970s. He got his first job hand-pressing Diane von Fürstenberg's signature purple shadow. He colour-matched it and won the business, and that's what put him in business in beauty.

My mother is an iconic, striking woman – very graceful, mixed-race, green eyes. It was the 1980s, so she'd be wearing heavy eye make-up and a red lip. Being in New York, seeing the world around me and having that personal reference in the home made an impression on me.

MAKE came about when I had been working with the influential British designer and creative director Faye Toogood in various capacities. I reached a point where I wanted to do something that brought together different parts of my background. I was interested in branding and graphics and strategy, as well as making things.

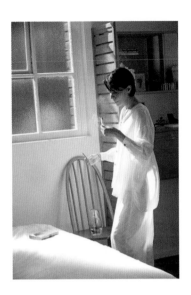

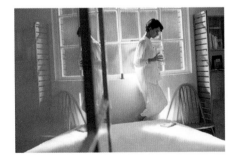

It was during the 2008 banking crisis, when Greece and Cyprus were going through a really difficult time. My dad wanted to find a way of using the business that made him successful to bring a wider vision of beauty to the world. His idea was to set up first MAKE, and then a series of brands that would all have this philanthropic aspect of supporting women-led cooperatives.

I never connected with the concept of a beauty girl. I didn't like how the industry projected its visions of beauty and what that looked like. I thought that often it reduced women to a skin-deep cliché. I felt there could be different ways to aspire to and connect with the beauty products in our lives. So when we launched MAKE, it was nice to try to create a different way to talk about beauty and to allow people to explore it in a new way.

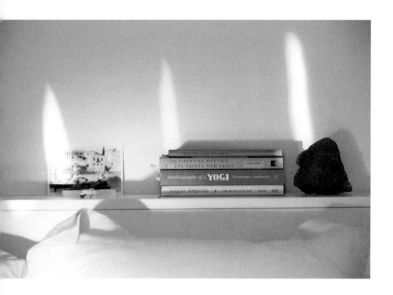

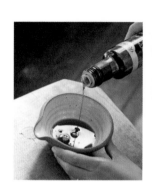

'I never connected with the concept of a beauty girl. I didn't like how the industry projected its visions of beauty and what that looked like.'

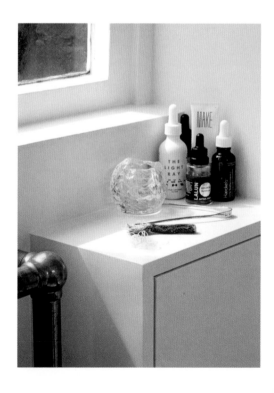

The idea for my ritual space, Cosmic Cosmic [launching in 2022], came about in a very personal way. I was going through a journey of grief and self-enquiry and trying to create new meaning in my life. When I left MAKE and began developing the idea for the space, I found many retreats and opportunities outside cities to do this soul-searching and journeying. But I felt the most important place to be able to cultivate this connection to oneself and one's practice was in the everyday. I felt called to create something that would feel like a retreat, but in an urban environment.

I want it to feel like a home, where you can come in and have a one-to-one conversation about different practices, or take classes – anything from meditation to movement, nutrition to life drawing or ikebana flower arranging. I'm also developing a line of products for contemporary ritual, which will include objects for meditation and self-practice and eventually personal-care items.

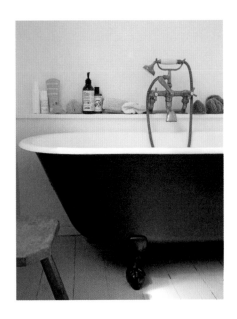

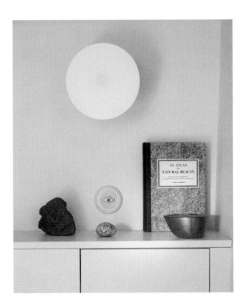

If I meditate in the morning, I look ten times more radiant than from anything I put on my skin. It's about that balance, learning to sit with my energy, let stuff pass, to start my day. That way of fine-tuning my frequency. Everything else comes after that.

I usually make a turmeric latte variation daily. Currently I'm making them with tigernut milk, Mariage Frères Iskandar green tea and a Bach Flower Remedy mix I've made with wild rose, oak, sweet chestnut and hornbeam. I sometimes add a rose elixir that I made with some dear friends, as well.

My personal beauty aesthetic evolves as I get older, but a go-to is always Audrey Hepburn. Her signature brows, clean, minimally made-up face and short crop were boyish and becoming. I was blessed with thick, dark Mediterranean hair, but have fallen into the cycle of my eyebrows having gaps and being uneven. Whether this is hormonal or stress-related, I have been trying my best to fastidiously remember to apply cold-pressed castor oil.

'For any beauty routine, for things to be effective you have to commit to them. Give them time; don't layer too many things. You're not going to wear five serums; they're just going to clog your pores.'

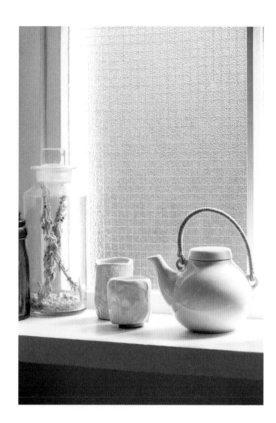

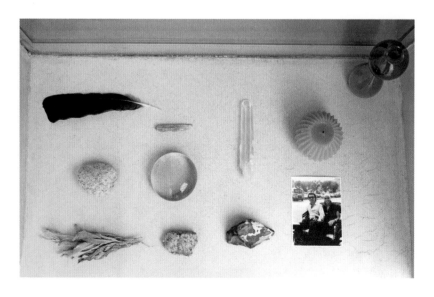

As the mother of a toddler, my 'routine' is ad hoc at best. Mornings start with tongue scraping and chewing on what my Jamaican grandmother called a 'chew stick', a vine or root used to clean one's teeth. I then floss and wash my hands with Austin Austin's Palmarosa & Vetiver hand soap. I spray or swipe my face with rose water, followed by my favourite Succulent Skin Gel from MAKE boosted with prickly-pear-seed oil from a cooperative in Morocco.

For any beauty routine, for things to be effective you have to commit to them. Give them time; don't layer too many things. You're not going to wear five serums; they're just going to clog your pores. The products I have the most of are my MAKE Succulent Skin Gel and body oils. They're multipurpose and nourish the skin. Hydration is the basis for healthful skin.

A favourite beauty destination is Buly 1803. What they do is incredibly charming. On my desk I have their book, *An Atlas of Natural Beauty*, a bible of different botanical ingredients for beauty. I like the way they look to different essentials across time and traditions, and the way they present everything, from the packaging and the calligraphy, which they write, to the sponges from Japan, and brushes and combs. I like the combination of objects alongside personal-care products – just things that you feel are good quality and will last.

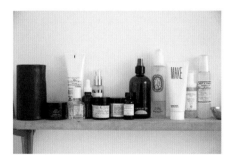

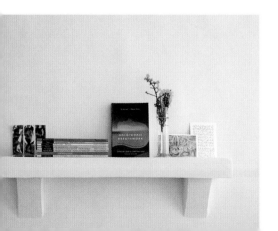

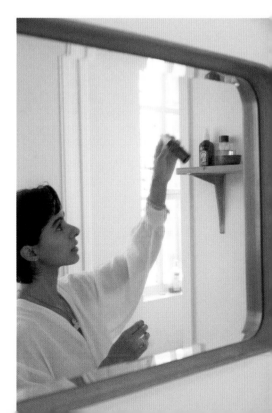

The Rituals:
Skincare

When it comes to skincare, it's complicated.
Really. When did it all become such hard
graft? I'm old enough to remember the
days when the 'cleanse, tone, moisturize'
mantra was more than enough and SPF was
a figment of someone's imagination.
We've come a long way.

Today skincare has almost become a competitive sport with
its panoply of essences, lotions, sleep masks, sheet masks, lip
masks, hand masks, not to mention an alphabet of acids and
serums. And yet it seems to me that there are more cases of
acne, rosacea and other skin inflammation than ever before.
Or are we just talking about it more?

Skincare is certainly a fashionable subject, and for that we
must thank the South Koreans, who are at the forefront of
pop culture and all things cutting-edge tech. 'K Beauty' (the
catch-all term for Korean beauty) is responsible for the
multi-step routines now popular in the West which promise
permanently bouncy, blemish-free, glass-shiny skin at every age.
But that has brought with it problems of product and ingredient
overload that in many cases upsets the skin's microbiome, its
natural pH-balancing ecosystem.

To go back to basics, skincare often starts with our
emotional state. According to Charlotte Ferguson, founder
of the psycho-dermatology skincare brand Disciple, there's a
proven link between skin health and mental health. Her own
psychotherapy research has observed the vicious circle of the
social media quest for perfect skin. The enhanced portrayal of
so-called flawless skin can lead to obsessive skin picking, which
she considers a form of self-harm: 'It can become addictive
because people get a release when they skin pick. They feel like
they've really cleansed their skin, or purged.'

In her psychotherapy practice Ferguson found that in many of her clients with anxiety, depression, low mood or trauma, existing skin problems were exacerbated during tough times. Her research found that stress triggers the 'fight or flight' hormone cortisol, which thickens sebum on the skin, leading to blocked pores and breakouts. To remedy this, her Disciple products use a variety of plant extracts such as ashwagandha (Indian ginseng) and turmeric to lower the production of cortisol in the body.

My takeaway from all this is to incorporate relaxing, tactile rituals into your daily skincare to help calm the mind. Start with a cleansing oil, which works by dissolving the oil in make-up, while nourishing rather than stripping the skin. Cleansing balms do a similar job and are especially suited to the night-time cleanse because they gently remove make-up (including eye make-up), sweat, sebum and sun protection without the

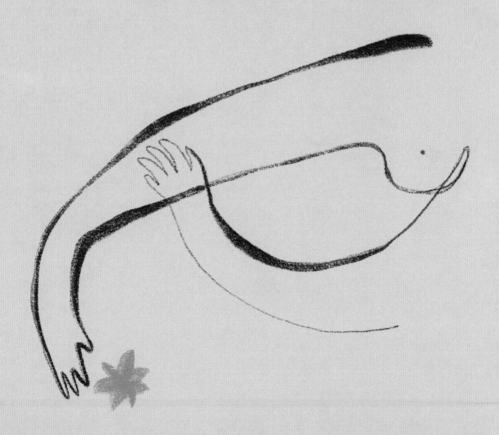

need to scrub. Just melt a little balm between the fingers and massage it into dry skin. This process feels extremely satisfying and nourishing, especially if there are added aromatherapy oils that you can inhale to help you decompress. (A note of caution: some people are allergic to aromatherapy oils, so avoid these if you have any skin sensitivity.) Then just emulsify the balm with a little water until it turns milky, and remove it using a warm, damp flannel or muslin cloth.

Oil cleansers are fine for oily skin, but if you have oily skin and find the idea somewhat terrifying, creamy rinse-off cleansers are equally therapeutic. Liz Earle's Cleanse & Polish is a classic, and the super-rich ones that come in a tube from Shiseido and Sensai have the consistency of old-school shaving balms – a little goes a long way. If you wear make-up regularly, follow the oil or balm cleanse with a mild foaming cleanser. This 'double cleansing' step removes any last trace of make-up and cleanses the actual skin underneath. Contrary to popular opinion, not everyone needs to cleanse in the morning. If you don't use make-up or much night-time skincare, you might find that a splash of water is enough.

After cleansing, moisturizing is my 'thing'. As far as I'm concerned, you can never have too much hydration, although needs can change according to age, time of year and climate. I like rich moisturizers in the colder months, such as the pharmacy favourite Weleda Skin Food from the German plant-based brand. But most of the time, a light glycerine moisturizer with collagen-boosting peptides, ceramides and hyaluronic acid will do the job. CeraVe Moisturizing Cream is a good option. In humid cities, try the refreshing gel formulations by Clinique and Glow Recipe.

As we head towards middle age our skin loses elasticity, causing dryness and wrinkles. This is of course completely normal. We can throw money at the problem with surgery, Botox, LED light therapy and injectable fillers, or accept it to some degree while committing to feeling as good as we can. 'I don't think you can reverse time. What you want is the best-looking skin you can have in your twenties, thirties, forties and so on,' says Victoire de Taillac-Touhami, co-founder of the French natural beauty brand Buly 1803. 'If you treat your skin well, of course you

might have wrinkles, but you can have good skin, even
with wrinkles.'

The subject of anti-ageing is nothing if not contentious, and
I worry that the pressure to have eternally peach-plump skin
causes unrealistic expectations. Instead, my tactic is to ramp
up the facial oils and face massage. No, they won't re-scaffold
the face, but they can have a temporary lifting and rejuvenating
effect that has the added bonus of feeling pleasurable to do.

As a child, I would be called on to massage my dad's face every
evening, kneading out the knots in his brows, cheeks and jaw.
To this day I view massage as an expression of love. After the
night-time cleanse and moisturize is the perfect time to do
some soothing facial massage. Nadira V. Persaud, make-up artist
and author of *Press Here! Face Workouts for Beginners*, recommends
a few minutes of brow-pressing or frown-knuckling exercises.
These increase blood flow and release muscle tension from
the vertical grooves in the glabella, the part of the forehead
between the brows. Simply place the knuckles of your index
fingers between your brows, press firmly and glide upwards in
short strokes, alternating between the left and right knuckles.
Or try using the Chinese Gua Sha tool, a flat, curved implement
made of jade or rose quartz, to sweep around the facial
contours. With regular use, this encourages lymphatic drainage
and the production of collagen and elastin. A rose quartz roller
can be similarly therapeutic. Use it as the beauty writer Saleam
Singleton does, to set you up for the day. 'It gives me a ten-
minute opportunity to meditate on myself in the morning, work
in my serum, do a little bit of skin sculpting, and just close my
eyes,' he says. 'It's another means for me to centre myself.'

Cleansing, moisturizing and holistic massage aside, there's a
world of treatments, serums, acids and peels out there. For less-
is-more ritualists, these can be overwhelming. If you're new to it
all, start slowly with weak concentrations of active ingredients
and gradual applications. Certain treatments, such as exfoliators,
which remove dead skin cells, leave the skin vulnerable to sun
damage. These are advised for bedtime, with sun protection
a must for daytime. Tread carefully and your skin barrier will
thank you.

Saleam Singleton

BEAUTY WRITER AND
CONTENT CREATOR

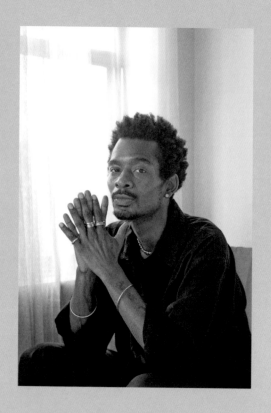

The beauty writer and content creator
Saleam Singleton grew up in Philadelphia with ambitions to
work in public relations. A love of media production piqued
his interest in YouTube, leading to his current mission:
amplifying the conversation about male beauty, mental health
and self-care. Now based in Brooklyn, New York, he is a
contributor to Byrdie Boy, and has set his sights on taking his
platform, The Method Male, to a wider audience.

I was always interested in media and film, so it was natural when I got into college to gravitate towards public relations. When I started to express myself and look for ways to explore products ten or so years ago, I was looking to YouTube, and I didn't see a lot of Black men. I felt a responsibility to create the media that I wanted to see. Now I'm working for Byrdie as a contributing writer for its Byrdie Boy franchise, starting a conversation with men in the beauty space.

My goal with The Method Male is to write more about beauty, culture and the intersection of race and self-expression. I am beautiful. Black men are beautiful. I don't think there should be some insinuation about a man's sexuality because he not only feels beautiful but also wants to maintain that beauty, inside and out. Skincare is merely an expression of that act of self-care that even today is very radical and brand new for Black men to express publicly.

I grew up poor. But through media, art, anime, movies and TV shows, I was able to survive, because I saw myself as a Black anime character. That helped me to see myself as something more. Even as an adult today I quite honestly see myself as an anime character. I love fashion and style, but I like a uniform. I was always taught that you should build a mythology around yourself and give people pictures when they see you, which should always be the same. That comes from my childhood, just seeing myself as a character in a story.

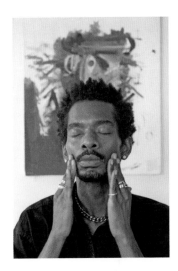

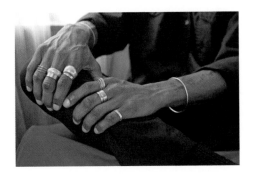

Mental health is extremely important to me. It's something that centres me as a man. Prioritizing it allows me to continue to perform in the spaces in a very genuine way because I know that I'm taking care of myself first. It's a combination of therapy and being able to communicate honestly with my family about my moods and feelings.

The first thing I do is cleanse. That's important because I use products at night and I want to get rid of that build-up straight away. When it's muggy and humid in New York I use Susanne Kaufmann's antibacterial cleansing gel to keep the breakout germs from my pillow when I'm sweating at night. I cleanse, tone, use a light serum and then a mist that can lock in the hydration. Of course I do sunscreen. I've been using Shiseido Clear Stick for years. It doesn't turn me purple, there is no white cast, and it works for all complexions and skin tones.

I really like using the rose quartz face roller because I'm a spiritual person and I believe in the spiritual influence of stones. It gives me a ten-minute opportunity to meditate on myself in the morning, work in my serum, do a little bit of skin sculpting, and just close my eyes. It's another means for me to centre myself.

I absolutely love fragrance. I love going to the Muslim shops and buying oils, but I also like my fragrances. Right now I love this company called Waft, which lets you design fragrances online. One of my all-time favourites is Thierry Mugler's Angel, the women's fragrance. I love being a man, I love being able to present as a man and express myself as a man. However, I do find a certain level of gender fluidity in my soul and in the way I love to express myself.

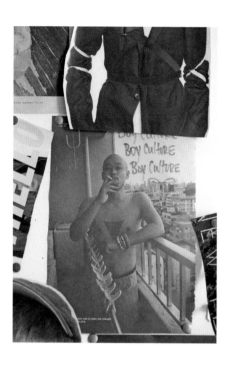

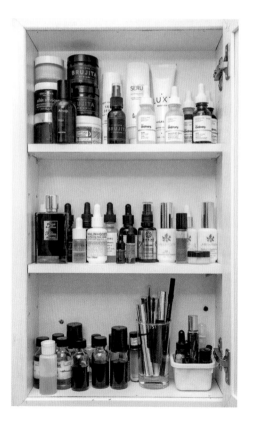

I think we're going to see a larger normalization of men expressing themselves through products in the beauty space. In terms of inclusion and diversity, I think we will start to see a more sincere reflection of men of varying skin tones and textures, and hair textures. Beauty is going to be what modelling and fashion were in the 1990s; it's going to become a part of pop culture.

I look forward to doing what I'm doing now on a much larger platform, and representing men who are ageing and men who are older. I don't think the scope of what is considered beautiful should just look like 22-year-old white guys. My ultimate goal is to have a show. I'd love to be like a one-man *Queer Eye,* to come in and have conversations with men and really explore the psyche, not just the product side of men in beauty.

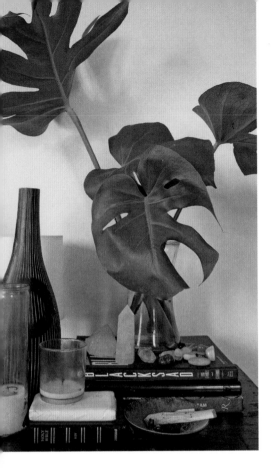

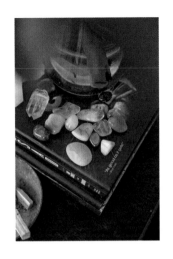

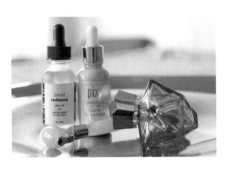

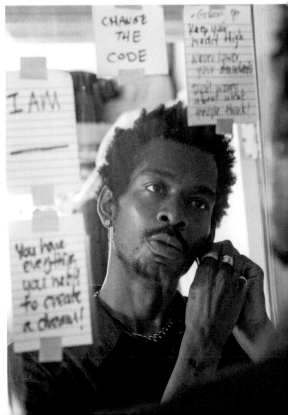

Susanne Kaufmann

OWNER OF BEAUTY AND SPA BRAND

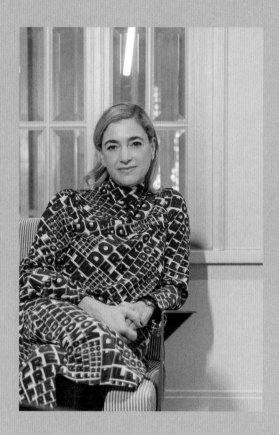

Turning her parents' Austrian hotel into a spa
was the catalyst for Susanne Kaufmann's pioneering
sustainable skincare line, SUSANNE KAUFMANN.

I was brought up surrounded by nature, in a culture where taking care of your skin, hair and body was of the utmost importance. My grandmother used to rinse my hair with camomile. It was a two-hour weekly ritual. To this day, nature is the cornerstone of my skin and wellbeing philosophy. Marrying the beneficial properties of Alpine flora with proven skin science is key to supporting the skin, so it can work at its best.

In Austria we have very deep roots in a sustainable and holistic lifestyle. This means that if you stay healthy, you feel and look better. Beauty is about being comfortable in your body. The skin is the body's largest organ and the 'mirror of the soul' – if one feels bad, one sees it immediately in the skin.

When I inherited Hotel Post Bezau from my parents, I very much wanted to embrace the beauty and healing power of the regional herbs and plants so beloved by my grandmother. For this reason, I made it my mission to create a modern destination spa that combined the natural bounty of the Bregenzerwald with a strong focus on treatment results and efficacy. My idea was to create a space where wellbeing took centre stage, placing prevention as the focal point of health. In 2003 we launched our brand SUSANNE KAUFMANN, with a curated range of 24 skin- and bodycare products.

'Beauty is about being comfortable in your body. The skin is the body's largest organ and the "mirror of the soul."'

Whether it's a hug from a loved one which makes us feel happier and more positive, or a massage from an expert which realigns our posture and improves blood circulation, the power of touch boosts both our physical and our mental wellbeing in many ways. This comes down to a connection, a value that is important for us as human beings.

The power of plants should never be underestimated. To ensure that we do not lose any of the strength nature has bestowed on our ingredients, we use cold-press extraction when obtaining the plant oils and compounds. It's a unique way to extract the very best parts of a plant and retain its potent bioactive properties.

Exercise is a very important form of self-care for me. Twice a week I go for a run or bike ride in the mountains nearby. Two or three times a week I take a Pilates class, or go to our fitness room and work with the weights. And lastly, baths. They are a great form of self-care. This was my inspiration to develop so many bath products in the SUSANNE KAUFMANN range.

Linda V. Wright

BOUTIQUE OWNER

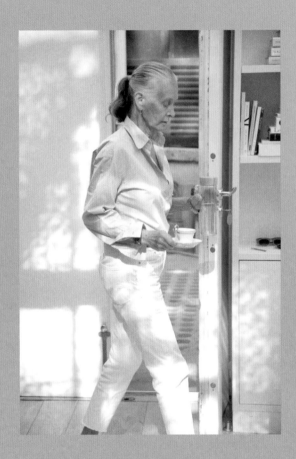

Born and raised in West Texas, Linda V. Wright was
led by an early modelling career to a love of Paris. Now
based in the City of Light as the owner of the classic knitwear
boutique Crimson, she delights in welcoming visitors from
around the world, while dispensing life learnings and style
advice to her faithful Instagram followers.

West Texas women are known to be of forceful character. I was born and raised there, among the cotton fields, dust storms, rattlesnakes and ranchers. Thus I naturally inherited a certain willingness to make something out of nothing. When I was 24 I made my first trip to Europe, and it was during this time that I fell in love with Paris. So, when I was 30, and at the very end of a modelling career in the USA, I felt it was time to try something new. That was 42 years ago.

My childhood was extremely difficult and there was never enough money except for the bare essentials. I mention this so that you will understand that dreams need hard work to come alive. Do not let them be lost as a passing thought without the action needed to make them become your reality.

I do feel that wellness equals beauty, and not the other way around. Obviously, this is such an individual and intimate routine for each one of us. I find that the beauty industry and the many products available have become overwhelming. I am a more than willing participant in this ever-expanding business of beauty products. I can't help myself!!! I love trying a new cream or a new serum. However, the information is endless, and I am still searching for those products that simply work for me.

'Make-up is non-existent in my bathroom. I prefer a nice clean face with my skin looking nourished. The glow is the goal.'

I have my speech prepared when approaching the consultant on a skincare stand. It goes something like this: 'Hello, I am hoping you can help me. As you can see, I have spent far too much time in the sun and I have what is referred to as mature skin. At the same time, my skin is problematic and prone to redness and dryness. Do you have a miracle product?' After a little laugh, we get down to business.

I always opt for the richest creams available in any skincare line. A major factor – and one that is a bit tedious, but makes all the difference in the performance of a skin moisturizer – is the massaging that assures the absorption of the cream. I start my massage at the neck and work my way up to the forehead. I also knead the cream into my skin. Think of kneading the dough while making bread and work the cream into your skin in the same manner. This increases the blood flow and gives my skin a certain glow.

Make-up is non-existent in my bathroom. I prefer a nice clean face with my skin looking nourished. The glow is the goal.

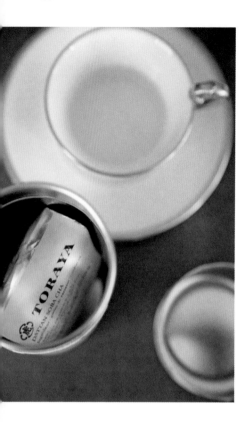

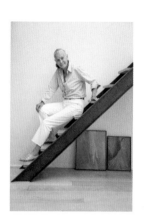

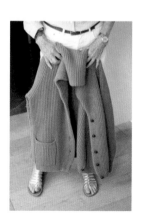

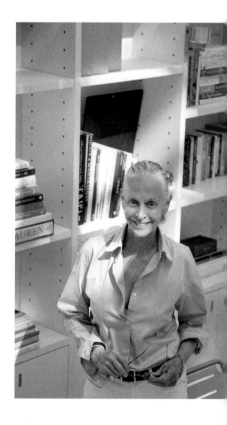

In September 2017 I had a transient stroke after a flight from San Francisco to Paris. My neurologist explained to me that I had created the accident myself, since my exercise routine had taken a back seat to me showing up early in my boutique. Stress had taken the place of meditation, and drinking a litre of water a day was non-existent. So, now I have a morning exercise programme and I do not allow myself excuses to skip. It's never too late to turn your life around.

My problem with perfumes is that they have always given me an immediate headache. But I have found my ultimate solution: Jo Malone's body cream in Nectarine Blossom & Honey. This is my most treasured moment every morning.

I had my last fling with blonde hair when I was about 50 years old. My hairdresser in Paris – David Mallet – said, Let's have some fun. So we cut my hair very short, dyed it white, and then I let the grey grow in while continually cutting until it was all natural. I have never looked back. I love when I can run my fingers through a healthy head of hair. Leonor Greyl's hair products are the best. There is a fabulous choice of shampoos, moisturizers and masks.

I must admit that I am a bit confused about this whole anti-ageing campaign. Why deny yourself the pleasure of accepting yourself at this age and relaxing a bit? In the end it is all about quality of life at any age. Ageing is a privilege denied to many people. Respect your age, young or old.

I am constantly trying different skincare lines, and I change regularly. However, I do not give myself permission to try something else until I have wiped the last dollop of that cream out of its jar. I will admit to loving those little sachet samples. I always say yes! They are great for packing when travelling. I look like a child in front of a candy counter when the consultant is placing them in my purchase bag.

I love having the first early morning hours to ensure a certain good energy level for the day. Breakfast consists of my favourite buckwheat tea that I buy at Toraya, my preferred Japanese tea salon in Paris, and some fresh organic fruit or a piece of gluten-free toast with honey. Afterwards, there is a quick change into exercise mode and concentration for a one-hour home-grown exercise programme. This consists of some stretching, upper-body muscle-toning exercises with light weights, working on the ever-difficult middle section of my body and finishing with a sun salutation.

Running my boutique, Crimson, is a full-time job, but I love communicating with those who are kind enough to accompany me on my Instagram journey. I rely on this particular social media to help me convey the messages that I feel are encouraging. If I were to be completely honest right now, I should admit that my goal is to help ladies of a certain age feel happier with themselves. Technology has given me the opportunity to reach out and give them a hug and some help.

I no longer buy anything for my personal skincare regime that is presented in a plastic container. This is one of the latest in my conscientious decisions to help clean up this planet for the next generations. We must all be involved. End of story.

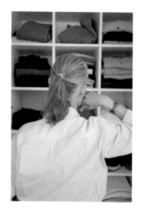

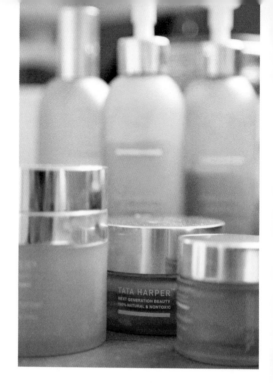

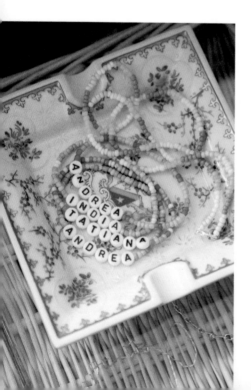

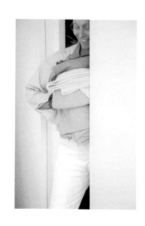

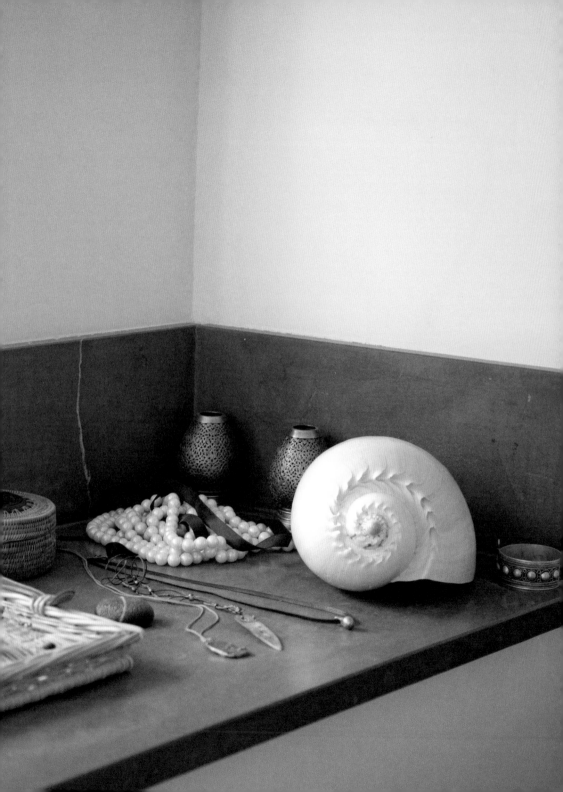

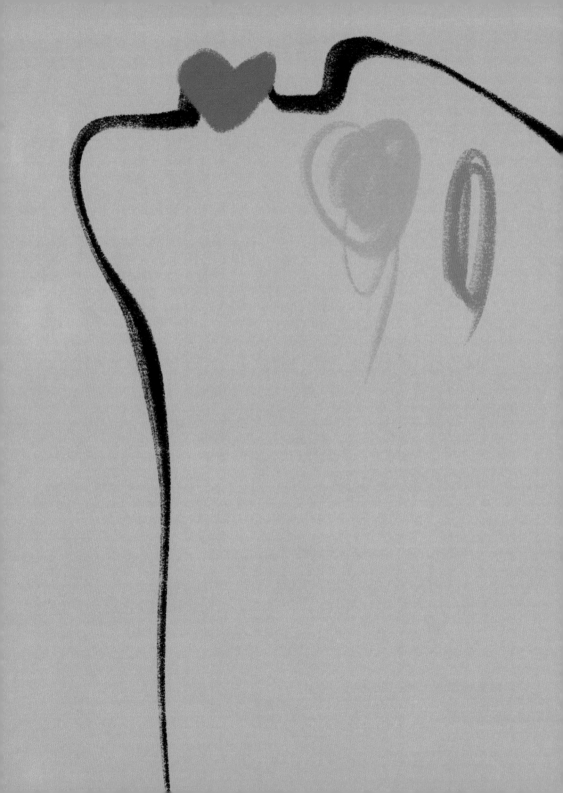

The Rituals:
Make-up

As the next generation becomes better informed about good skincare, will there be less need for excessive camouflaging and 'perfecting' in the future? One lives in hope. 'Skin should look like skin,' says Gucci Westman, a make-up artist and founder of the beauty brand Westman Atelier. 'My signature make-up look is super naturally dewy skin where you almost wonder if it is or isn't make-up. The glow that comes from dewy skin just projects good health and wellbeing.'

Of course, therein lies the paradox. Good skin shouldn't 'need' make-up, but many of us like to have an element of enhancement and enjoy the process of putting it on. Even if it's barely there 'no make-up make-up', the act of applying it is pleasurable and feels transformative. The concentration required is meditative, even when the result is as minimalist as an Alex Katz canvas.

Make-up formulations have evolved so much that it can be hard to tell where skincare ends and make-up begins. But the key is always to prep the skin properly before application. Westman likes to exfoliate gently first, then pat on a hydrating serum before using a facial tool to help lymphatic drainage. (Try simple facial massage to help with this, too.) After adding moisturizer, she applies her highlighter stick on the tops of cheekbones, at the inner corners of the eyes and above the Cupid's bow, before applying foundation or concealer. These are subtle enhancements that you can't really get wrong if you apply with a light hand.

The secret to understated make-up lies not so much in the number of products you use, but in the textures and application. While the job of foundation is to even out the skin tone, remember that skin is rarely one uniform tone. Apply a balm-like foundation, such as Westman Atelier's Vital Skin, in sheer layers only where needed. Another tip is to leave the bridge of the nose foundation-free for the most natural effect.

Texture-wise, dry skin responds best to moisture-boosting foundations. Look for the new-gen formulations with added skincare benefits such as hyaluronic acids, peptides and ceramides to keep the skin hydrated but groomed throughout the day. Alternatively, add a drop of facial oil or serum to your foundation – this is also a great way to dilute it for lighter coverage.

For oily skin that's prone to breakouts or shine, water-based foundation is less likely to clog pores. Or look out for the new oil–water hybrid formulations, such as Chanel's Les Beiges Water-fresh Tint. This futuristic gel contains pigment-filled oil droplets that merge to leave a weightless veil on the skin. This is a great option for teens, men or anyone who wants to look groomed but not visibly made up. On that note, the men's counter is a good source for make-up minimalists. Ranges from Tom Ford, Boy de Chanel and Shakeup tend to be tightly edited and geared towards fuss-free application.

As with foundation, less is more where concealer is concerned, and it should be as invisible as possible and melt into the skin. For undereye circles, first tap on a lightweight moisturizer (or eye cream) to create a smooth surface for the concealer. When it comes to the minefield of shade matching, the make-up artist Shinobu Abe offers this basic guidance on undertones for foundation and concealer: 'Most people have a yellowish undertone, except those with very pale skin, who tend to have a pink undertone. Mid-brown complexions usually have an orange undertone. And those with darker, Black skin tones suit a red-based foundation to avoid looking "ashy" and bring their skin to life.' In Japan and Korea, where the overriding beauty ideal is still 'pale is better', there's a tendency to choose whitening foundations. 'Not only is that an outdated beauty ideal, these pink-based foundations are simply the wrong undertone and look completely unnatural on Asian complexions,' Abe cautions.

We're living in the age of 'glow': luminescence, vitality and dew-dusted cheekbones. The easiest way to add that summer-in-Saint-Tropez *bonne mine* effect is with highlighter balms, cream blushers and gel bronzers, applied with the fingers. A small amount of bronzer blended where the sun naturally hits the face – the tops of the cheekbones and the temples, plus a tiny amount added to the eyelids – is the easiest five-minute face you can do. Translucent, iridescent balms can be blended with coral cream blusher to create a natural-looking cheek tint.

If your make-up goal is subtle enhancement, skip the supersized eyeshadow bricks for individual cream-to-powder pots or stick pencils. The most versatile are dark neutrals: browns, khakis, maroons and taupes, perhaps with the tiniest hint of iridescent shine. I also really love an eye gloss that can be worn alone or on top of a powder or cream-to-powder shadow for a very relaxed, casual look. Add a little brow gel and mascara (top lashes only is fine) for more definition.

Finally, to end on a cliché, if you have only one lipstick, make it a red one – it's the universal smarten-upper that suits everyone. 'You put your red lipstick on, a little mascara and it gives you that extra boost you need,' says the London wellness coach Isa-Welly Locoh-Donou. 'You're clean, you look great, you feel great, you present yourself and people are attracted to your aura.'

Marie Humbert

ACTOR

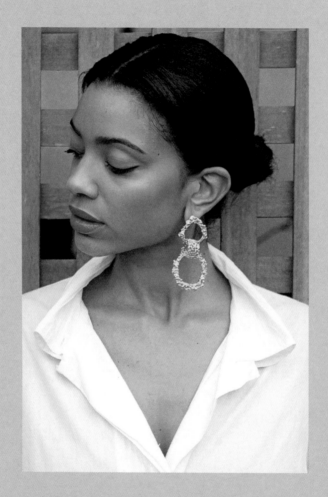

Swiss-Ghanaian Marie Humbert is an actor, connector and champion of the arts. Passionate about nurturing Ghanaian talent, she supports local beauty entrepreneurs, but also delights in the wonders of humble plant remedies.

Beauty for me is to be as natural as possible.
I mean, I love make-up, but my father always told me,
'You're not supposed to look like you have make-up
on. Just use it to enhance the little things about you.'

**There was an acting opportunity in Ghana and my
mum said I should come and try it out.** I thought,
why not? So I auditioned for a web series called *An
African City*, which became quite successful and was
dubbed by CNN and the BBC the *Sex and the City* of
Africa. It's a representation of Afropolitanism: these
women who are independent, powerful, unapologetic,
who aren't the stereotypical representation of an
African woman. She's not afraid and she doesn't
need a man.

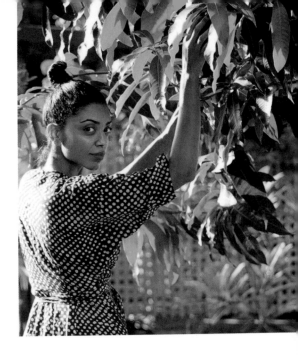

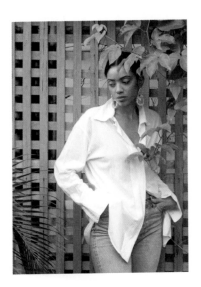

**As much as it's fascinating to take on a role, it's
also quite scary** as you fully delve into the life of
this character. Regardless of the role, it's always a big
responsibility and a rather intense journey.

**While in Accra, I realized how much of a vibrant
city it is, bursting with emerging talent.** I looked
around and was like, what more can we do to support
young local artists, creating more platforms that allow
them to share their talent and ideas but also learn and
be inspired? So I created an event called Cocktails
Over Fashion with the main objective of inspiring,
informing and challenging creative minds. As the
title suggests, it is now focused on African fashion
designers but eventually I want to include more
members of the African arts and culture scene.

**I'm not a very kind person before coffee in the
morning.** Hot water and lemon? Nobody's got time
for that. It's cute, but no. I need my coffee; I function
better after that. I wish I could say I meditate and
chant, but I haven't yet found that app! I practise yoga
and try to be as active as I can. I don't deprive myself
of anything, it's all about moderation for me.

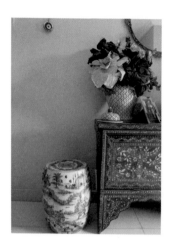

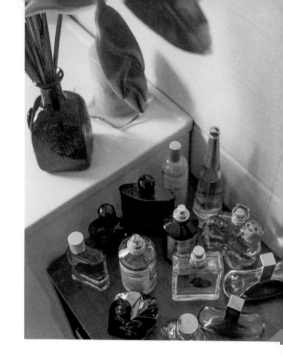

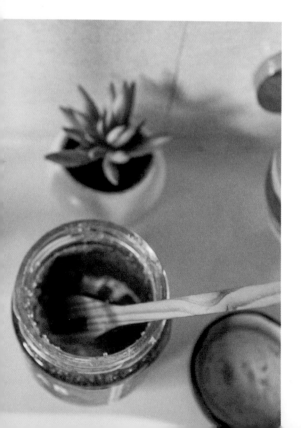

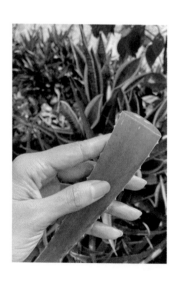

I'm passionate about supporting oils and products from Ghana. For my body, I sometimes wash with natural black soap from Ghanaian brand Skin Gourmet, blended with either peppermint or raw honey. I also use their organic facial scrubs with coffee or moringa. I love to moisturize with 79 Lux balm. I live for organic baobab oil, raw shea butter and aloe vera from my garden, I use all head to toe!

My make-up is very simple. I apply a little MAC concealer, I've never been a foundation person, but I like Bare Minerals loose powder foundation. Then I fill in my eyebrows with my MAC pencil, and I always put on mascara. I have two moods, either a bold eye or lip, never both together, but the bold lip is usually what I go for.

'I'm not a very kind person before coffee in the morning.'

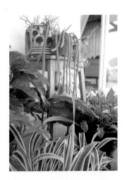

I'm not very experimental with my hair. My ritual in the morning is to sleep for as long as I can, then I usually tie it in a bun. Recently, I've enjoyed braiding it in really long braids. I sometimes blow-dry and straighten it, but I'm mostly very easy with it.

The education my parents gave my brother and I was focused around strengthening our sense of identity. My mum is Ghanaian, my father is Swiss and we lived as expats around the world so it was important to them that we know and love where we are from. As a result, we never allowed anyone to tell us who we were or where we belonged, that was only for us to decide and no one else. Every day I thank my parents for that, I realize now that I'm much older how incredibly important that was.

I'm very aware of my emotions and my feelings, I wish I could protect myself better sometimes but that's an ongoing process. I do acknowledge when things are overwhelming and when I need to take a break. Self love is a process.

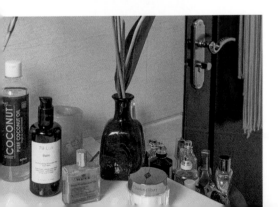

Bethann Hardison

FASHION ADVOCATE

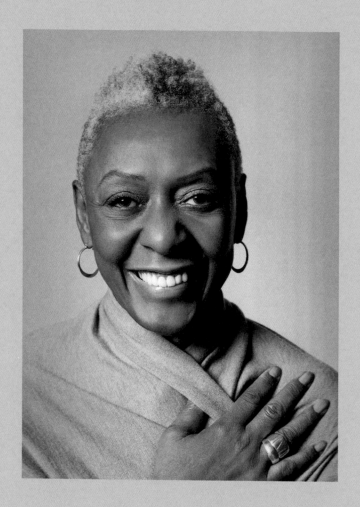

The mission, by fashion advocate and
former model Bethann Hardison, to celebrate
models of colour helped to transform the fashion
and advertising industries.

I grew up in a neighbourhood where everyone had some sort of style. I was always interested in how clothes are made and how they get out to people. I wound up getting a job at a custom button factory, where the owner sent me out to deliver the buttons to the design companies. I then went to work for a junior dress designer. And then the designer Willi Smith discovered me. He thought I was a designer because he'd seen me in the garment district. I became his muse.

My first runway show was for a merchandizing executive called Bernie Ozer. I went up to him and said, 'You know, if you want to have a great show, you'd have me in it!' I created the Black Girls Coalition in the late 1980s to celebrate so many models of colour beginning to work. That was the great move of Regis Pagniez, who was sent to New York from Paris to start American *Elle*. And thank God, because he just saw girls he liked, and they were of colour, so they started to work more and more. I was a model agency owner by then, and because I was a Black owner too, I related. We were teaching the girls how to use their celebrity, in a very smart way.

'I created the Black Girls Coalition in the late 1980s to celebrate so many models of colour beginning to work.'

By 1996, once I'd closed my model agency and moved to Mexico, the models of colour disappeared. Eastern Europe started to open up and casting directors wanted nondescript girls who all looked alike. Ten years went by and I did my first press conference, to defy the notion that that was all right. It had to stop. In 2007 Franca Sozzani published the all-Black issue of Italian *Vogue*, which helped to change the perception of the girl of colour.

Now these girls are working, they're all shades, all colours. But the real objective was to see how I could affect society's visual mind, because that was my remit, something I knew well, that industry. People would instead notice colour as being very normal, because once you start seeing it, it doesn't seem such an odd thing. Now the only thing left to do is to get more people of colour who can do the jobs behind the scenes as well.

My rituals? I love to try to have a hammock everywhere I live! I'm someone who likes to go for scrubs, massages and saunas; I love to space out in heat. I stretch every night and day, because the body needs limberness as you get older. I don't have to do a lot of caring for the skin. Most of it is totally inherited. But I do cleanse at night if I've been out in the city, in the elements. I will take a cleansing cloth and wipe my face, and put a little bit of facial oil on my skin. That's it.

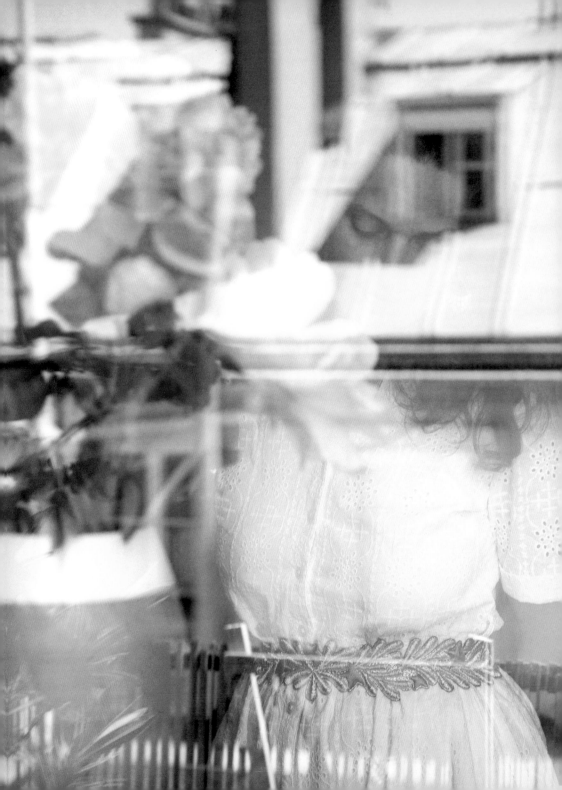

Victoire de Taillac-Touhami

CO-FOUNDER OF
BULY 1803

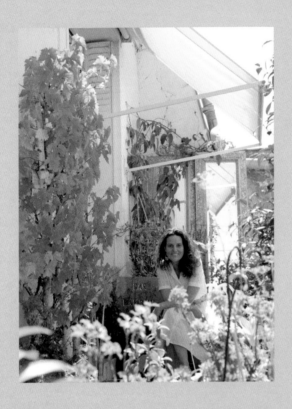

Starting her retail career at the age of 22 as PR for the cult Paris concept store Colette, Victoire de Taillac-Touhami discovered a passion for beauty. With her husband, Ramdane Touhami, she went on to launch Buly 1803, revamping an ancient apothecary for a modern audience. An advocate of herbal remedies and global rituals, she published *An Atlas of Natural Beauty* in 2018. At her home in Paris, her bathroom with its bath salts, balcony and 'wardrobe of oils' is her sanctuary.

I was born in Lebanon, in Beirut, because my parents were working there, but during the civil war I grew up in Paris, so I'm a Parisienne. At university, my best friend was Sarah Andelman of Colette. She was going to open a store with her mother, Colette, so I joined at 22 and stayed for six years. We were very young and free, so we tried everything. Colette was so dedicated, so passionate about what she was doing; it was the best training to work alongside her. That was how I discovered that I prefer beauty to fashion.

When Colette opened, they wanted to bring in things that were not available in Paris. We had the first Kiehl's counter outside New York. The department stores were very old-school, so brands like this were all trying to get into Colette to enter the French market. Then, I decided to do my own thing with my husband, Ramdane. We opened the first niche beauty store in Paris, Parfumerie Générale. This was really the beginning of my relationship with retail.

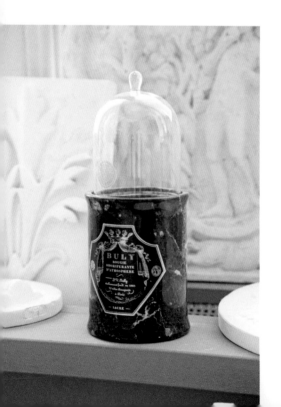

In my family, beauty was sophisticated and very simple. The interest was more in terms of lifestyle – healthy living or what you should eat. My interest in herbal beauty came from Dennis Paphitis at Aēsop, because when we launched the brand at Colette, the training was really very serious, carried out by Dennis himself. It was two full days, and very plant-orientated. Afterwards, because I love to eat, I really got a sense of the wellbeing benefits from plant-based products because you become very sensitive to the quality of good ingredients.

I use very few beauty products a day, but I'm really obsessed with hydration. I love the Dieter Rams idea of 'less and more', and that you should be very precise about what you try on your skin and just take the best. I love it when I'm in a Buly store and I hear how creative people can be with their whole beauty routine. It's very personal, and that is what I like.

I'm a big believer in dry body brushing. I always use a German dry-brushing brush. My morning routine is either dry brushing or a cold shower, depending on the day. Then afterwards, a lotion and maybe a raspberry-seed oil, and then a body lotion on my skin. I don't like to see beauty as torture, or as a competition. I'm not interested at all in being younger or thinner; I just want to feel good in myself.

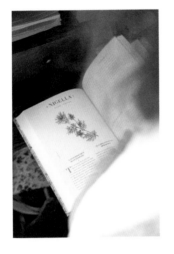

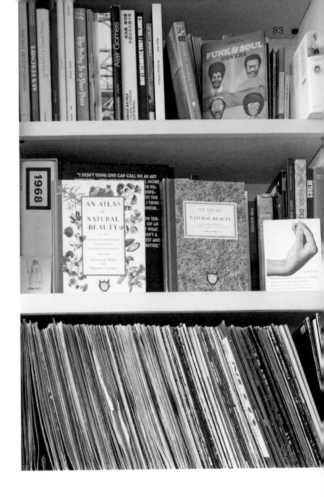

'Japanese stores are the best
in the world, in terms of service
and display. It's a very, very
sophisticated country for beauty
and they're mad about skincare.'

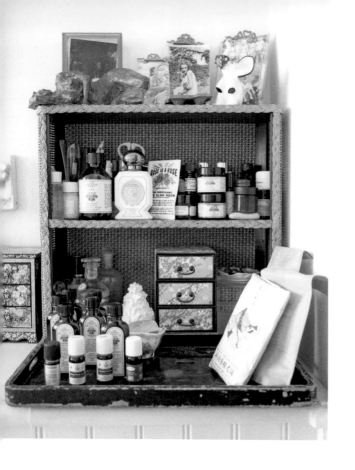

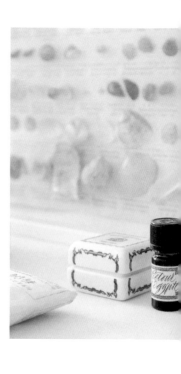

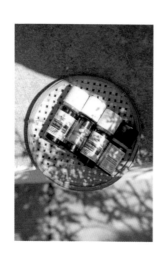

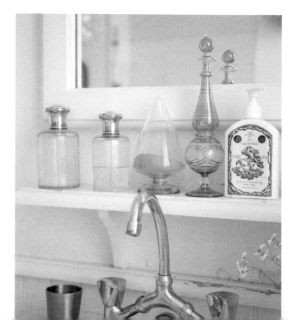

Oral care is not only about brushing your teeth. I love the copper tongue scraper, which is genius when you don't feel great. You really have the feeling that you're very clean after cleaning your tongue. I also love oil pulling. It's disgusting: you have oil, which you swill around inside your mouth, and it takes with it all the bits that are stuck, and afterwards you just spit it away. When we started working on the toothpaste for Buly we were quite surprised at how difficult it was. It's so complicated, so expensive, but I think oral care is really important.

At Buly, we wanted to revamp this historic beauty brand and give Paris very beautiful beauty stores. We wanted, when the customer enters, for them to be able to find anything, from perfume to oil to a beauty accessory; we wanted a dedicated beauty store. It's like going back to the roots of what a beauty store used to be. You can buy a rose perfume or rose cream, but you also have access to rose-petal powder because the culture that I love was all the things you were doing at home for yourself. We're very passionate about beauty secrets from around the world.

Water is a big thing in my life. I love a hot bath, closing the bathroom door and nothing else can happen; it's like leaving the outside world from your bathroom. I'll put all sorts in the bath, from Epsom salts to essential oils or whatever I have. If I'm into it I'll do a mask at the same time. In Japan my favourite beauty thing is onsen bathing. And in Morocco, the hammam is my favourite thing – fun! I enjoy that feeling of extra cleanness you have from these traditional beauty routines that involve water.

We love Japan. Japanese stores are the best in the world, in terms of service and display. It's a very, very sophisticated country for beauty and they're mad about skincare. They're very specific and knowledgeable about beauty. It's a very rich culture, and each time you go you discover something you hadn't heard about.

As I get older I notice that I enjoy scent in everyday life. The scent you don't expect, when you walk around the city and there's this amazing floral scent and you have to look to see which garden or balcony it's coming from. This is something I really like. I love to be surprised by smell; it could also be perfume on a friend. I love the freshness of cologne.

My worst habit is not using sunscreen. I don't even talk about it! I think it's been created to make you feel you need it, but there are many ways to protect yourself, maybe not going into the sun. I haven't used one for 15 years. Unless you take me on to a beach at noon and I can't move; then of course I would need to use something.

Our bathroom is a shared family bathroom, so it's quite messy. It has huge windows and a little balcony. I have a small cupboard and a kind of wardrobe of oils that I like for my hair, face and body. I like to unwind in my bathroom, so I like to have nice things in there, a few objects, some candles or a drawing.

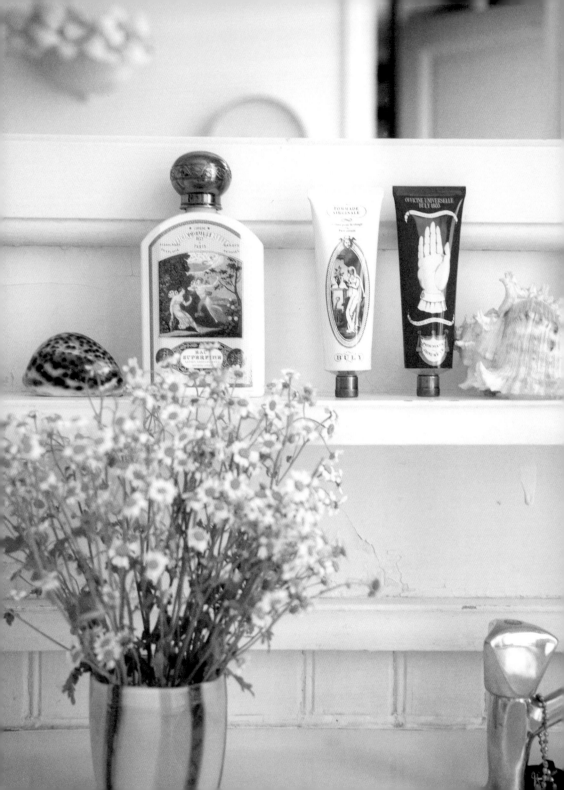

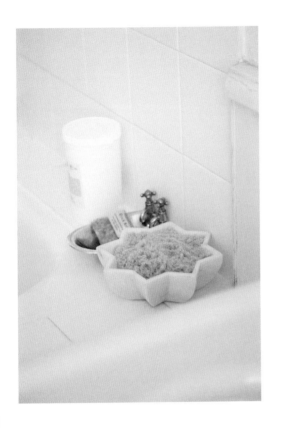

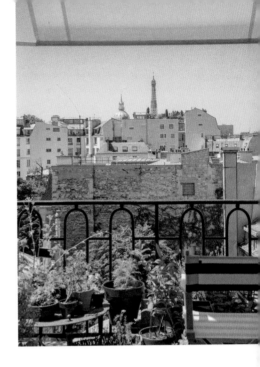

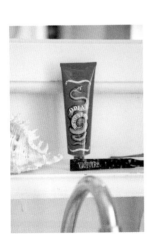

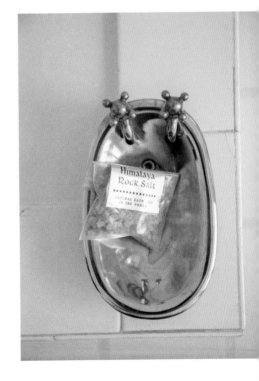

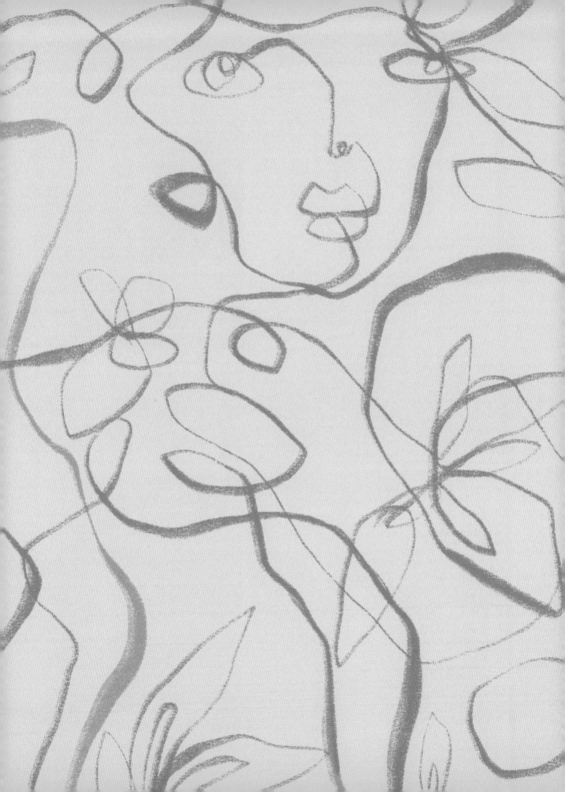

The Rituals: Fragrance

'There's so much visual stimulation now. A baby's sense of smell is its most developed sense. It can find milk by smelling. But we don't use our sense of smell, nor have the education to develop it,' says Ryoko Hori, who runs scent workshops in her Berlin salon, Senses. Here she focuses on the 'lost' senses, giving visitors the opportunity to experience different fragrances and the emotional connections they evoke.

It's true that we live in a visual world. If you want to see, listen to or taste different things, there are endless options for places to visit, but if you fancy exercising your olfactory 'taste buds', you're limited to a perfumery, perhaps, or a garden. That's a shame, because our olfactive senses are extremely powerful. Scent and emotion are located in the brain's limbic system, which is also connected to memory. This explains why certain smells have transportive emotional associations – a kind of aroma therapy, if you will.

Recent developments in neuroscience have allowed perfume companies to look at scent that breaks down cortisol, reducing stress and stimulating the release of endorphins, the 'feel-good' chemicals produced by the brain. Brands are using aromachology – the study of how smell affects behaviour – to create mood-enhancing products that also make us smell great.

Hori flags the ritualistic elements of scent in producing feel-good micro-moments. She notes that for centuries candles, sandalwood and incense have been used in ceremonial and spiritual practices to connect the present to the past. Fun fact: the word 'perfume' comes from the Latin *per fumare*, 'to smoke'.

'I remember the smell of incense from my grandmum's house, as well as sandalwood and ouds,' says Hori. 'They remind me of my memories. It's calming. Incense came from China to Japan and was very much a spiritual ritual and a way to communicate with ancestors. During an incense ceremony in Japan, they don't say "smelling", they say "listening". Listen to Buddha, listen to your condition.'

Burning rituals aside, wearing perfume is a way to express or evoke a mood, and the process of applying it is in itself a transformative ritual. I gravitate towards light colognes when I want to feel energized; the refreshing citrus notes of bergamot or lime give the senses an instant wake-up call, even in midwinter. For a warmer, more sensual mood, seek out the rich notes of tonka bean, oud woods and animalic musks. The most intense ones, such as Nasomatto Pardon and Frédéric Malle Musc Ravageur, have an almost intoxicating effect, so are best applied sparingly.

In recent years we've become much more experimental in the way we wear scent, realizing that clichés such as gender and occasion are imposed by marketers. Niche brands are overtaking the beauty giants, and having a single signature scent has given way to a more mix-and-match approach. This applies not only to the smell but also to the vehicle. For example, if the alcohol component irritates your skin, try wearing one of the

Scent is a hugely important factor of self-care, both in the ritualistic burning of oils and candles and in its stress-busting powers.

many perfume pendants or solid balms containing perfume oils that are now available. Hori's own alcohol-free powder perfume is another option, inspired by Japanese rubbing incense, while the boutique owner Linda V. Wright swerves traditional perfume altogether in favour of Jo Malone's Nectarine Blossom & Honey body cream. 'This is my most treasured moment every morning. It nourishes my skin and gives just the slightest hint of perfume that everyone seems to notice,' she says.

You could also consider crafting your own perfume. Once available only to the 1 per cent, bespoke perfume has become more accessible, with workshops such as the Experimental Perfume Club allowing entry-level alchemists to concoct something original. Alternatively, the perfumer Maya Njie suggests simply combining a spritz or two of your own complementary favourites to create a scent that is unique to you.

Scent is a hugely important factor of self-care, both in the ritualistic burning of oils and candles and in its stress-busting powers. Aromatherapy is rooted in the practices of ancient China, Egypt and Greece, though the term itself was coined only in 1937, when the French chemist René-Maurice Gattefossé discovered the healing benefits of essential oils. The oils were also used to disinfect and heal injuries during World War II.

While aromatherapy has long been dismissed as modern-day snake oil, improvements in regulation and the quality of ingredients have boosted its credibility. Fuelled by the success of brands such as Aromatherapy Associates, This Works and True Botanicals, the industry is now projected to be worth US$9.57 billion by 2026, taking it out of the 'alternative' bracket and firmly into the mainstream. This can only mean more and better products coming our way. As sleep and health are the new totems of luxury, pillow sprays and de-stressing rollerballs are the new It accessories. Try breathing in a wrist-full of This Works' Stress Check rollerball before an interview, or a deep inhalation of a lavender essential oil-soaked hankie before a flight. Or, to decompress after a busy day, sniff a sprig of lavender from your balcony pot plant to achieve the same effect for no cost at all.

Arpana Rayamajhi

ARTIST AND JEWELLER

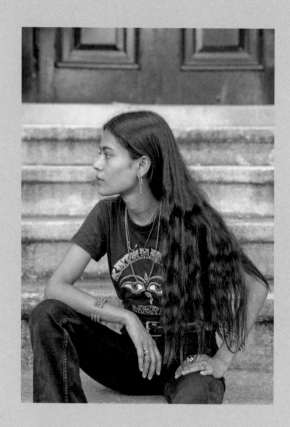

Born and raised in Kathmandu, the artist Arpana Rayamajhi was inspired by the natural grace and style of her late actress mother. After creating music in her home country, she moved to New York to study painting and sculpture. She now studies acting and designs jewellery that expresses her deep-rooted love of colour. To help her deal with city life, she relies on a green tea habit and hydrating rose masks, and takes pleasure in the pain of a deep-tissue massage.

I've been attuned to beautiful things ever since I was a kid. I was always fascinated by actresses and actors, childishly comparing them and wondering which one was prettier than the other. I wasn't aware of the beauty and modelling industry when I was a kid because I grew up in Nepal. The culture there was completely different. Young women, regardless of how beautiful they were, could not make a living just being pretty.

I was forced to think about my health and mortality when my mum was diagnosed with cancer ten years ago. She had already overcome a lot to become an actress in Nepal, and ended up taking care of two of her girls after my dad passed away. Yet she would still always dress up, do her hair, and at least put on a dab of lipstick. Just seeing that somebody appreciates beauty and curating things around herself despite her trauma, she's probably my only real inspiration. I'm a cliché: my mother inspired me!

'I completely understand that we all want to feel connected to our roots. But it doesn't mean that we can't also be the perpetrators of maybe exoticizing ourselves.'

If I don't drink green tea in the morning, it's like walking out without necklaces or earrings. When my mum got unwell I started looking up various antioxidants that were good for you, and green tea seems to be one of the best.

The super-obsessive culture about identity is predominantly an American thing. What I've noticed is that oftentimes, it may come out of good intentions, and we tend to point the finger at others for doing something wrong with somebody else's culture. But at the same time, what some of us fail to see is that we ourselves are propagating this idea of a certain culture that actually doesn't exist back home. I completely understand that we all want to feel connected to our roots. But it doesn't mean that we can't also be the perpetrators of maybe exoticizing ourselves.

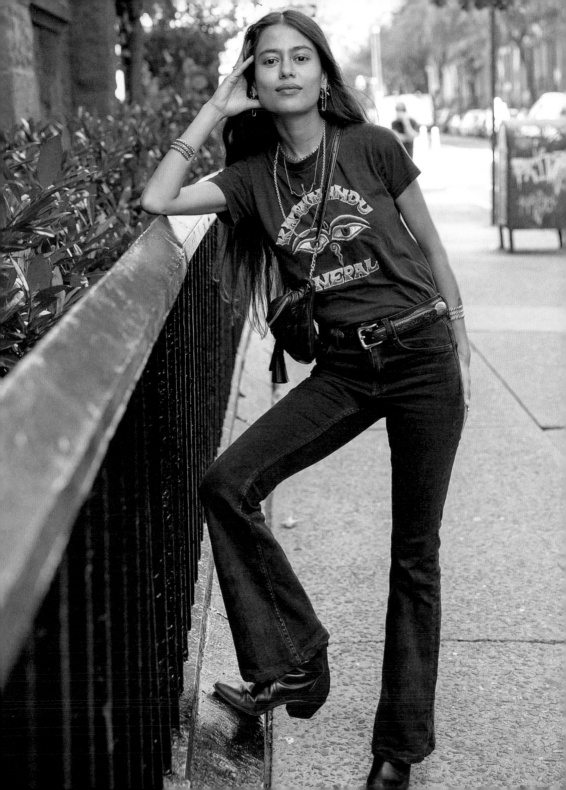

The one thing I'd like to do that I've never done and I'm kind of scared of is Vipassana. It's an intensive course where you basically don't speak, you try not to make eye contact with anyone and you don't do anything but meditate pretty much all day for ten days. I feel it would make me know myself better, know my limitations, where my emotions are coming from and how to handle them better.

I'm crazy about massages and acupuncture. I don't like anything too soft; I like feeling a little pain. I love a good deep-tissue massage. The masseuse makes it feel like they're taking care of you, and you're a little baby.

Nepalese women are really big into oiling. On my hair I use everything from olive oil to mustard oil, almond oil and amla oil, which comes from the Indian gooseberry. I just wash my hair with Japanese tsubaki shampoo and conditioner, which is really good for when my hair's frizzy, and then I air-dry it and apply the oil on my scalp.

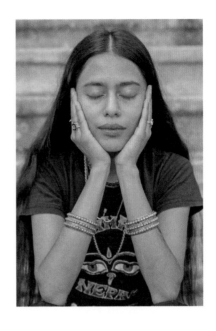

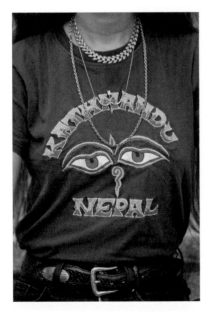

The one thing I'm obsessed about is skincare. Sometimes I think I can see all of me through that one pore! I think it goes back to having acne when I was young. And, can I say something? Often when women are pushing for no Photoshop, no retouching, I completely agree, but I also notice that the people pushing for no Photoshop have never had breakouts or don't have problem skin.

I love doing face masks. As much as I think there are some really good sheet masks, I think it's a bit of a consumerist twist to masks that already exist. It creates so much more garbage, and I don't want to incorporate that into my beauty. I do hydrating masks. I have a rose mask by Fresh that I do every once in a while.

Colour is strength and power where we come from. To enjoy it means you're alive. I like to wear animal-friendly lipstick, predominantly in pinks and reds. I wear Milk Makeup lipsticks and lip balms.

Gucci Westman

MAKE-UP ARTIST AND FOUNDER
OF WESTMAN ATELIER

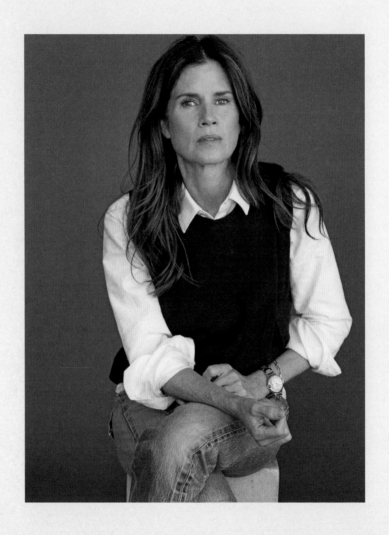

The make-up artist Gucci Westman's 'anti-perfectionist' beauty look and curiosity about ingredients inspired her make-up line, Westman Atelier.

I wasn't allowed to wear make-up growing up, so of course I rebelled and played with it! When I was 18, I became an au pair for the fashion journalist Anouk Ortlieb. She would take me to shows with her and share the boxes of make-up that were sent to her. Later I enrolled in the Parisian make-up school Neo Christian Chauveau, and then left for Los Angeles to take classes in special-effects make-up. I met Spike Jonze and started working on all these indie movies. I ended up meeting Annie Leibovitz and Bruce Weber, and started working with them. Bruce told [*Vogue*'s then creative director] Grace Coddington about my work and she hired me for two *Vogue* shoots – and then I got really busy!

I can't stand the over-the-top Instagram look. Skin should look like skin! As a make-up artist, I want to enhance features, not cover them up. There's this trend in the beauty world for the constant search for perfection. It saddens me to see how women and men view themselves today. Why can't we feel confident with just a little boost as opposed to such extreme transformations?

'Skin should look like skin! As a make-up artist, I want to enhance features, not cover them up.'

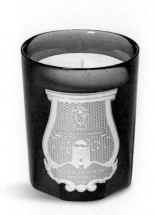

Developing rosacea was a huge catalyst for me when I started Westman Atelier. It's an incredibly frustrating skin condition – you never know what you're going to wake up to. It propelled my already curious nature about ingredients and healthy living to a greater focus on the ingredients we put on our skin.

I love natural scents that come from body moisturizers and oils such as coconut, vanilla and shea butter. Cire Trudon's Manon candle has been a favourite for years. The lavender scent with touches of sweet orange is so calming.

Honey Dijon

DJ AND CREATIVE

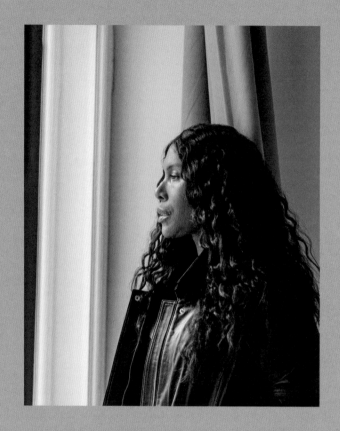

Growing up in Chicago during the emergence of house music, the DJ, music producer and trans activist Honey Dijon discovered her love of style through culture. Now based in Berlin, she has started to build her brand empire with a clothing line backed by Comme des Garçons. With a passion for feel-good rituals, wellness and plant-based cooking, she has set her sights next on beauty domination.

My parents were very young when they had me, and they liked to party a lot. They liked to get dressed up and my dad used to get a lot of shit in the neighbourhood, because he was quite non-binary at a time that was *super* binary. He used to wear clogs and tank tops and carry satchels, so I was really informed through my parents about the power of clothing and, if you weren't part of the norm, the effect that had on people.

I was born in Chicago at the beginning of the house-music culture. You had your own dialogue with the way you dressed to find your tribe. A lot of the time that was influenced by the new-wave scene that was coming out of New York, and also by disco. That was when I first heard about Italian and French fashion, because you had all these innocent kids wearing European designers to dress up and go to the club. That's how you spoke to other people who were into this music.

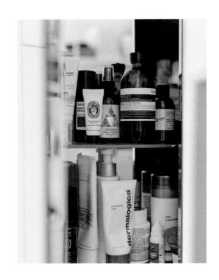

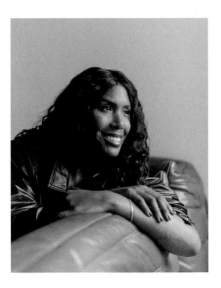

We lived in the suburbs, so I used to have to take a train into the city. There was this store called Wax Trax, where all the punk, new-wave, indie kids went. That's where I found out about *The Face* magazine, and *i-D* and *NME*. It was like all this bombardment of culture, music and art. The biggest influence on me was the fashion designer Stephen Sprouse. At the time a lot of kids were emulating what was happening in downtown New York. Lots of black, heavy eyeliner, lots of blown-out hair. Grace Jones's flattop was a huge inspiration among the Black kids.

Everything I've ever been attracted to has been reflective of culture. What's inspiring me in the moment being reflected in culture is the deconstruction of gender. This whole non-binary movement that's happening with the new generation, where it's not about men's clothing or women's clothing, men's make-up or women's make-up, it's just about beauty and how you choose to express yourself. It's a combination of body parts and gender expressions, beauty aesthetics and different areas mixed together. It's deconstructing my whole idea of what I thought beauty was.

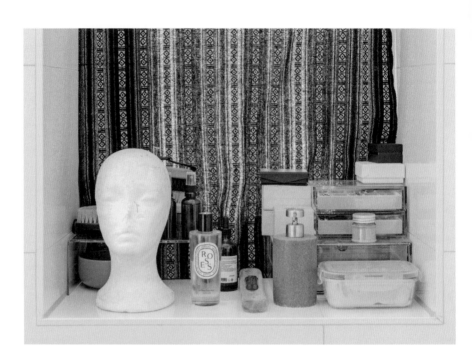

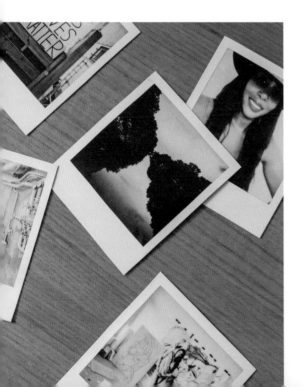

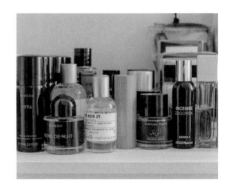

Even in the last five years we've had the diversity conversation, but the people from minority groups are still not the ones in power. Where are the trans and non-binary fashion photographers and editors and festival owners? One of the things I realized from my 'Honey Fucking Dijon' collaboration with Comme des Garçons is that I'm the first trans woman of colour to actually work with a major fashion brand, with my own name on the label. I get to express my vision and that's not being dictated for me by someone else. I think that's really powerful.

Wellness and beauty are intertwined. How you feel about yourself is really the ultimate beauty weapon: what you eat, what you put on your skin, the people you surround yourself with. I try to surround myself with people who uplift my vibration instead of squashing it. A lot of it comes from dismantling your belief system, what you believe to be beautiful and what is beautiful to you.

'Gendered fragrance is so old-school, you need to get over that.'

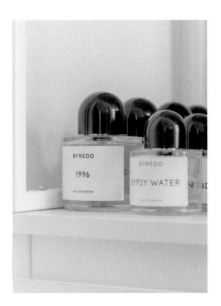

I had really bad skin when I was a teenager. I tried everything; I became a vegetarian out of vanity. I went down a rabbit hole of dry brushing and shea butter and sleeping and water and learning as much as I could about probiotics and gut health. And then going into yoga. I was really into wellness before it became commodified.

I just love oils. They're natural, they're healthy, and there are not a lot of additives in them. I love rose and patchouli; I guess I'm a hippie! I even wear perfume to bed. The pharmacy has a really great rosehip oil that I use on my face, and shea butter I get from Sun Potion. They make really great adaptogenic powders, too.

You'll also find Dr Hauschka skincare and Weleda Skin Food in my bathroom. And my dry-brushing brush and neti pot, because I use a neti pot every day. So I combine wellness with beauty.

My favourite make-up brands are NARS and Dior. I love that NARS is really about music and culture and art. I have to have an emotional reaction to something, and not just have it because someone says I should. It has to have a bit of substance and a story.

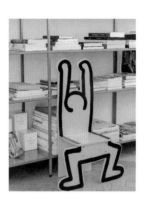

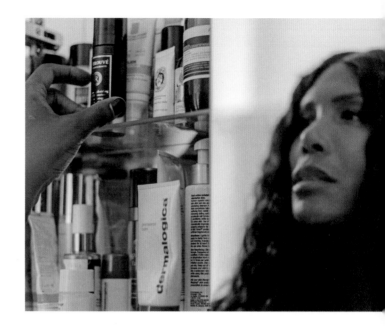

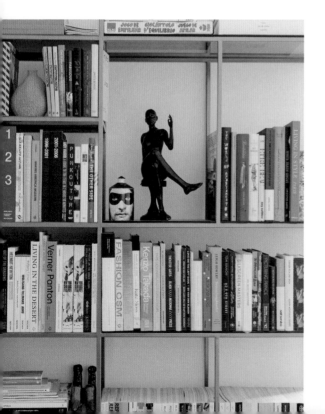

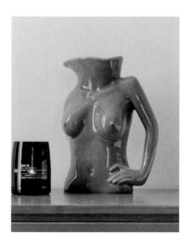

Gendered fragrance is so old-school, you need to get over that. It's really boring and it's really old. It should be about the beauty of the person, not about their gender. Genitals do not define gender, and shouldn't define your life story.

I remember more about how someone smells than how they look. Fragrance is very powerful, especially if you're falling in love with someone, or smelling a home-cooked meal. Every time I smell bread, or caramel, or vanilla, it reminds me of the warmth of my mum. I like to smell as good when I walk around every day as when I go to bed. It helps me; I like feeling sexy when I go to bed. I like feeling sexy all the time.

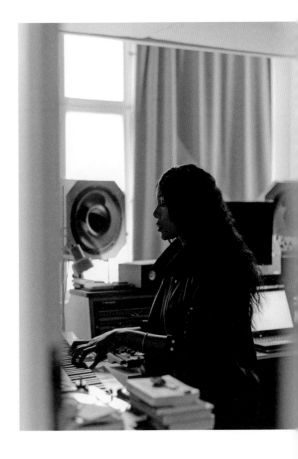

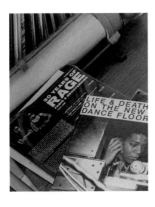

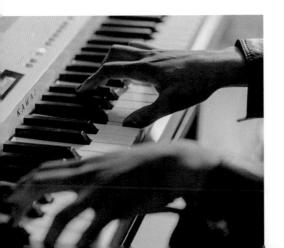

I'm obsessed with magnesium bath salts. I *love* bathing. It's one of the most beautiful rituals, with Byredo candles to de-stress. I have a lot of Palo Santo and incense that I do in the house. My meditation is a whole ritual. I like to mist, and I have my mantras that I do and then meditate. Mostly my mantras are full of gratitude for everything I have in life. I thank the universe for all the blessings I have, and ask for more!

My next step is to be the new Madam C.J. Walker [the legendary Black beauty entrepreneur and activist]. So, skincare and beauty. And eventually I want to open a canteen that serves really amazing plant-based food from a beauty perspective.

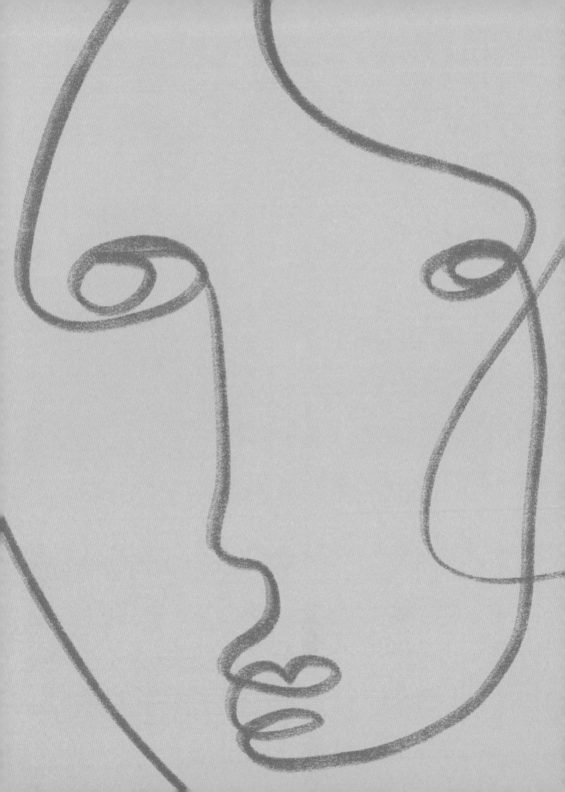

The Rituals:
Hair

Perhaps even more than fashion, hair is our most important identity signifier, communicating taste, politics and social standing without us needing to speak a word. After years of conforming to societal norms, it's experiencing its moment of self-expression. 'Hair is super-important, especially for people of colour', says the DJ and creative Honey Dijon, 'because we have taken something we've been oppressed with – our naturally curly hair – and made it an art form.'

For the perfumer Maya Njie, growing up mixed-race in Sweden and having Afro hair was a challenge because few products were available and nobody local knew how to work with her curl texture. The answer eventually was to cut it all off when she arrived in London, an act that proved liberating. Now, she focuses on scalp care using moisturizing jojoba, coconut and baobab oils with her own blend of bergamot, neroli and ylang-ylang essential oils to make it smell good.

In fact, the self-care for hair movement has gradually been gaining traction, with scalp care, brushing and conditioning taking on a less burdensome, more therapeutic role. Like skin, hair shows the effects of stress and hormonal changes, which are reflected in thinning, alopecia and lacklustre condition. Lifestyle habits can also affect it. If you're struggling with your hair, look at whether you're getting enough good-quality sleep, protein and relaxation in your life. Gua Sha, often used as a facial massage ritual, can also help to improve circulation in the scalp. For a daily boost, to drive nutrients to the follicles, place a Gua Sha comb in the centre of your skull at the front hairline and sweep gently backwards down to the neck, repeatedly.

Scalp scrubs and regular brushing are other pleasurable rituals that you can embrace to improve and maintain the wellbeing of your hair. Try the reviving scrubs by the Body Shop and Christophe Robin, and handmade combs by Crown Affair, a company created by its founder, Dianna Cohen, to make haircare more holistic.

For a long time society has forced women of colour to emulate Western hair while damaging theirs in the process. Flipping the switch on chemical straightening treatments, a new generation of brands has emerged to help restore the health of natural curls and coils. Curly hair needs moisture, something that sulphate-heavy shampoos end up stripping away. Newcomers include Pattern Beauty, Dizziak and Bouclème, owned by naturally curly-haired founders and offering products that use gentle ingredients to hydrate and treat.

Joining this trend are haircare brands such as Chāmpo (pronounced *shar-pour*, meaning 'to press and knead the muscles' in Hindi) that combine new technology with botanical ingredients to promote the Ayurvedic principles of mind and balance. This aligns with the trend for 'co-washing', a process that swaps shampoo for a conditioner with mild cleansing agents to clean and condition hair without depleting its natural oils. A great option for dry hair, it prevents the damage that can be caused by regular sulphate-laden shampoos.

As with skincare, a new entry to the world of Western haircare is the conditioning oil. While Westerners have a morbid fear of this all-natural substance, it's a much-loved secret weapon of many beauty ritualists. The artist and jeweller Arpana Rayamajhi learned about the advantages from her mother while growing up in Nepal, and continues the tradition: 'Nepalese women are really big into oiling. On my hair I use everything from olive oil to mustard oil, almond oil and amla oil, which comes from the Indian gooseberry.' The Japanese massage therapist Ryoko Hori also champions the power of oils. For her the magic ingredient is tsubaki oil, which comes from the seeds of the camellia flower. It's the oil that is used to give Sumo wrestlers' hair its incredible strength and shine. Try it as a calming leave-in treatment, working in a generous amount after towel-drying. Or go the everyday low-maintenance route. The Brazilian footwear designer Mari Giudicelli does very little to her naturally wavy hair, but after a shower she applies the traces of Costa Brazil body oil that are left on her palms to the ends of her air-dried hair.

It doesn't stop there. You can also consider the wonders of oil as an eyebrow- and lash-boosting treatment. The wellness coach Isa-Welly Locoh-Donou extols the benefits of humble castor oil: 'I put it on my lashes and brows before bed. I've done that for several months, but the lashes get silkier. I buy castor oil and put it in an empty mascara tube and add vitamin E.'

With all the talk about natural and holistic haircare, where do we stand on the (aptly coloured) elephant in the room? To cover up grey hair, or not to cover it up? Despite all the progress in the beauty industry, ageism is still rife, and costly dyed hair is considered standard. 'Hair speaks volumes about the confidence of a woman,' says the seventy-something boutique owner Linda V. Wright, possibly the coolest woman I know. 'Women become almost belligerent when discussing the decision to continue this ritual of dyeing their hair. Ladies, going grey and growing older is a privilege we should embrace!' Her tactics took her to the salon chair of David Mallet in Paris, who cut her hair super-short and allowed the grey to grow in, while continuing to cut it until it was its natural de-pigmented shade. She then tied her hair into a signature updo, aided by a choice of Leonor Greyl shampoos, moisturizers and masks: 'I have never looked back.'

Mari Giudicelli

FOOTWEAR DESIGNER

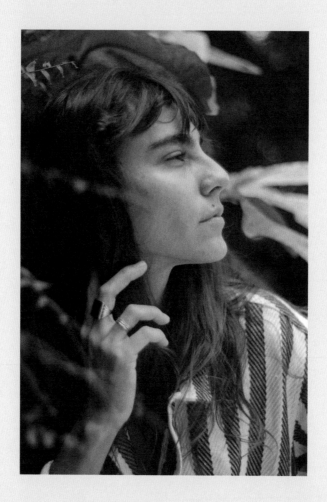

Growing up in a culture of impossible beauty
standards, Mari Giudicelli questioned the narrative.
Her low-maintenance, anti-perfectionist aesthetic suits her
laidback lifestyle – in New York an accidental footwear
entrepreneur, and in Brazil a sun-loving water baby.

I remember watching my mother getting ready in the mornings. She had long, wavy hair, and to me, that was the ultimate illustration of beauty and femininity. I grew up in Brazil, where there is a very strong beauty and body culture and a lot of pressure to fit in, have your nails always done, your hair tamed and your body hair shaved. This was introduced to me at a very young age through teen magazines, TV shows and friends at school. Eventually, I started questioning it, why do I want to have blonde hair, why do I have to have my nails done every week, it seems wasteful? What's really my perspective on this?

I've always been obsessed with Brazilian music from the 1960s and 70s, especially the women such as Gal Costa and Maria Bethânia. I love their looks and outfits, all very organic and sensual, with natural hair and sun-kissed skin. I believe less is more; I'm not into the idea that recently every girl's getting fillers and other procedures, ending up looking like the same person, or chasing one specific aesthetic. To me that behaviour supports unrealistic beauty standards that aren't very healthy.

I really don't do much to my hair. I did straighten and dye it many colours when I was younger, but today the less I do to it the healthier it feels, so I just let it be. I wash with shampoo every day and I rarely use a conditioner – only when it's super tangled – and I let it dry naturally. I use Costa Brazil oil on my body because it smells divine, and whatever's left on my hands I might put in my hair ends to add some shine.

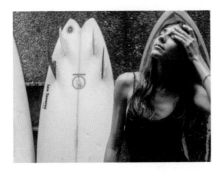

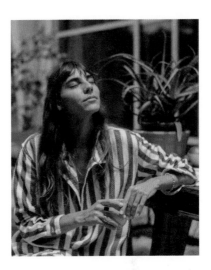

Like everyone else, I used to pluck my brows a lot. That required a lot of maintenance. I'm glad I started seeing beauty in big brows and that that is an essential part of me that I now appreciate.

I try to be practical and not spend too much time on my beauty routine. In the morning I usually just wash my face with warm water; then I use an ice roller to make me feel more awake and de-puff my face and follow up with sunscreen. At night I use a moisturizing serum and rotate between active creams.

I'm always swimming. I either go to the pool or to the beach, any body of water I can find. The mental and emotional part of swimming is the most beautiful thing to me. If I'm in the ocean, I feel extremely connected to nature, and that's one of the things I miss the most about Brazil.

I love Korean spas. I enjoy going on my own so that I can truly take the time to disconnect from the outside world and be present. I find it all very meditative and healing.

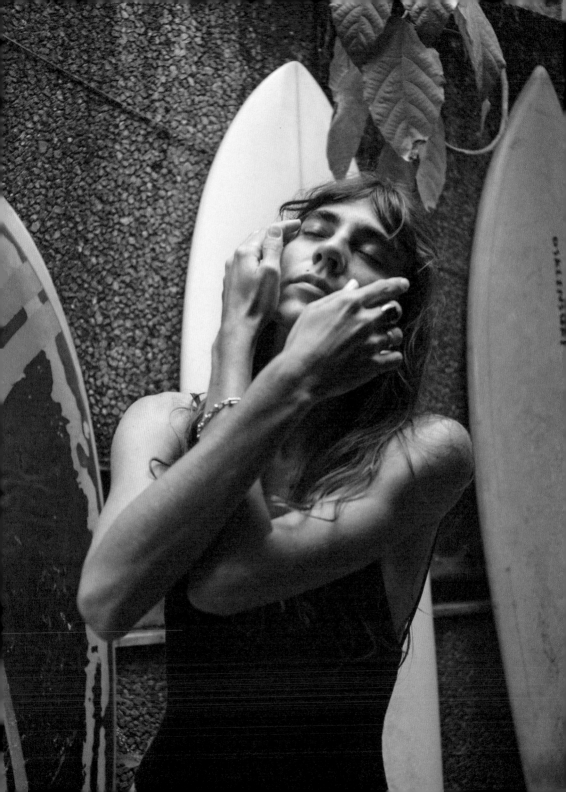

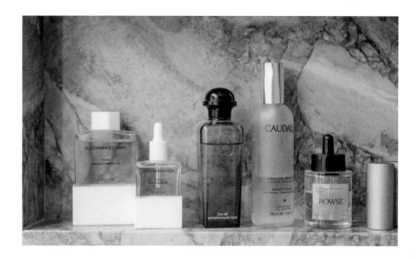

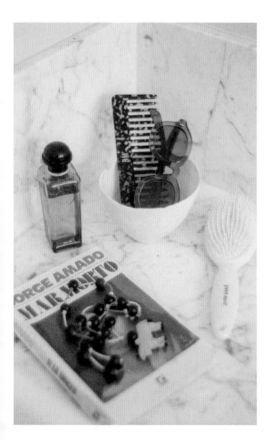

When I went into business as a footwear designer, all I wanted to do was make shoes, but over time I realized I needed to become a businesswoman. I started it when I was 25, and I didn't know what I was getting into. It is a daily challenge, I'm always learning. The newness of it is very exciting. It's about growing and being out of your comfort zone.

The beauty industry is very powerful. It plays off our insecurities and is a symbol of status. Being conscious about what you use and why is really important, instead of buying a product because the packaging looks nice. Our skin doesn't need ten products a day, it really doesn't.

I try to buy something new only when I run out of it. My relationship with beauty products changed considerably after I read a book called *Beyond Soap*, by Sandy Skotnicki, a dermatologist who is specialized in skin allergies. She explains that sometimes a natural product can be worse than a 'chemical' one. Hidden ingredients labelled as fragrance can be very bad for you. The goal is to use only 'clean' products. That's why you need to know what works for you and not buy something because someone else did. So my approach is more about finding products with ingredients listed very clearly on the packaging, so you know what is in it and if that's what your skin needs.

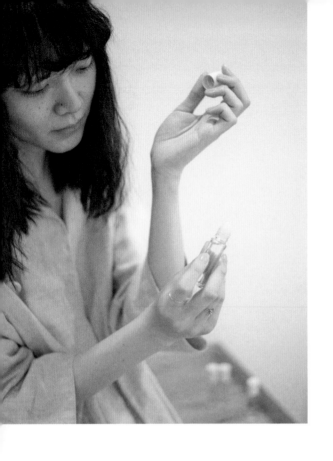

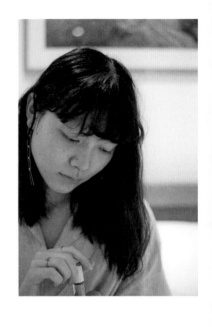

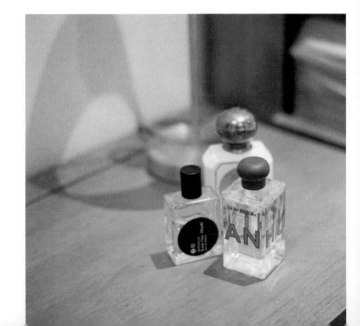

Taira

MODEL AND INTERPRETER

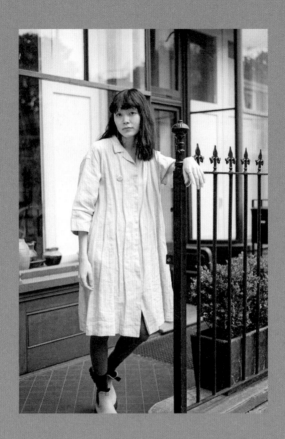

Hailing from Hokkaido, Japan, the model and translator Taira spent time in London reading cultural studies and semiotics at Goldsmiths, University of London. An interest in identity politics informed their outlook on modern Japanese culture and the role of gender stereotypes in society. Growing up in a family of doctors instilled in them an appreciation for wellness practices, from the Confucian idea of *hara hachi bu* to forest bathing.

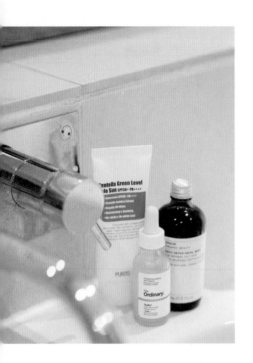

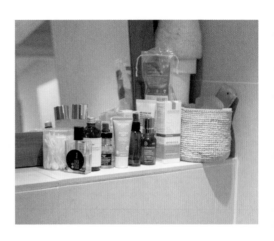

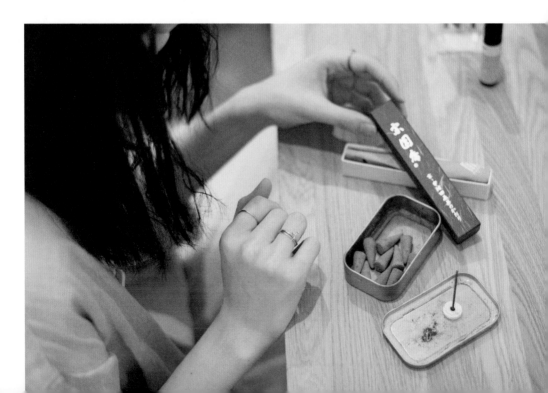

I am originally from Hokkaido, the most northern island in Japan, known for its food, nature, agriculture and farming. At Goldsmiths I learned a lot about gender, ethnicity and the politics of identity. It cultivated in me the desire to think about society and my intersectionality.

I think a lot about our aspiration to be beautiful and what it means to be well, or healthy. It sometimes feels like a quest that has no end. Discussion of those topics, especially when beauty is involved, can be quite empowering, but it is also a tricky subject to address. Where I grew up there's a very strong ideology around the type of standard that you should meet. If you do not follow it you would be seen as a failure, or a slacker who gave up the game.

I definitely sense more pressure in Japan towards people who identify themselves as female or women in general in the matter of beauty. There's so much expectation for them regarding the traditional gender norms, roles and body image. It feels quite patriarchal. When it comes to identity politics, Japan shouldn't be proud of where it's been. I constantly felt the pressure to blend into society in order to 'maintain harmony'. I guess I was forced to be self-conscious because of the strong peer pressure I felt and it was quite stressful to cope with.

I don't associate myself with any gender category. I used to have some preferred labels that I'd like to be identified with, but I felt I was differentiating myself from others, so I was othering myself by stating my identity, which did not sit right with me. So whenever people ask my pronoun, I let them choose, which often confuses them. But ambiguity is really important for me, and for the world.

I come from a family of doctors, so health has always been an important matter for me. School lunch is considered an educational opportunity in Japan, so the food is made from fresh ingredients to recipes created by nutritionists. We learned healthy eating habits, such as *hara hachi bu*, which means 'eat until you are 80 per cent full'. Chewing well is one of the things I learned, because we use chopsticks, which naturally helps us to eat more slowly and chew our food properly.

I wash my face with warm water; I don't use any cleanser in the morning.
I follow the steps I have from Japan, which are toner, essence and moisturizer. I like toner from Liz Earle, which is good for my sensitive skin. I like the essence from Deciem that has vitamin C and anti-ageing properties. For night-time I use Weleda Skin Food Light moisturizer.

I don't wear much make-up. But sometimes I wear subtle make-up just for myself, to feel good or to play with it. I like glowy-looking skin. I use Glossier highlighters and blusher that you can use for your lips and cheeks.

I have a cup of matcha tea every day for all the great health benefits and antioxidants. It helps me to stay focused and awake during a busy day. I tend to get a caffeine high from coffee, but I don't get it from matcha.

Modelling is like acting. It's a type of performance. I perform different versions of 'Taira' for that moment in time; it's like an exploration of identities, and I've been finding myself transforming every time, which I really enjoy. I personally think it is impossible for an individual to have only one identity, and in that sense modelling has taught me a lot about the performative elements of our lives. It allowed me to explore new ways to express myself to others.

'I have a cup of matcha tea every day for all the great health benefits and antioxidants.'

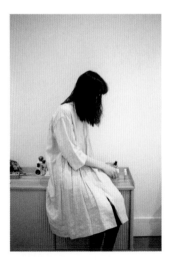

I've been into aroma since I was little. I used to love picking the bath salt for the day. I like gentle, tender scents, and I also enjoy changing fragrances depending on my mood. Most of the time I carry some fragrance roll-ons in my bag, or solid perfumes, to refresh my mind when I get stressed during the day. I like Jo Malone, and I've got some incense that I really like from Japan, so I've been using that a lot.

I like visiting mountains in my home city. So whenever I go back to Japan that's like my power sports. I try to make time to do some forest bathing, which is a Japanese ritual. It's not exercise or hiking or jogging, it's simply being in nature. It helps you to relax and focus on the present. I try to do that when I go to my home city, and just get away from the crowd without listening to music, without any digital devices, just enjoying what I hear in nature.

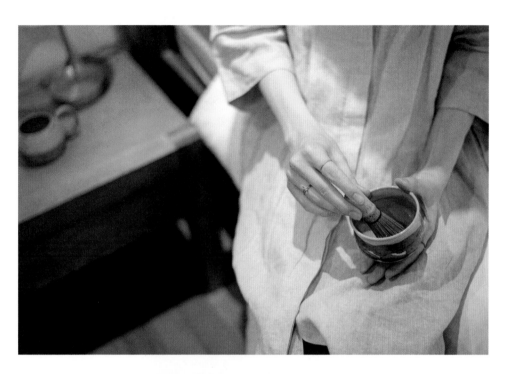

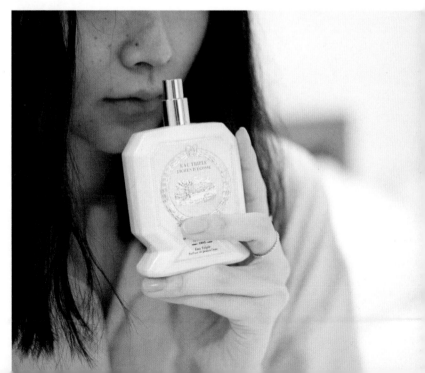

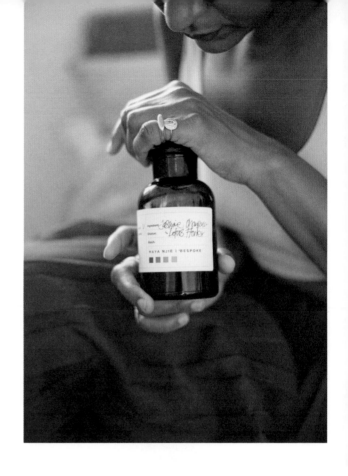

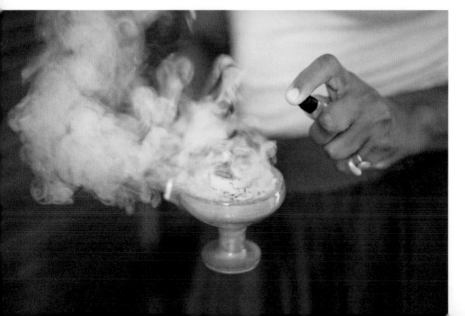

Maya Njie

PERFUMER

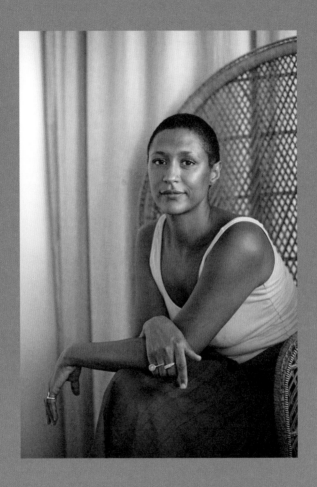

The Swedish-Gambian perfumer Maya Njie uses
her family photos as inspiration for her fragrance
business. Growing up in the Swedish city of Västerås,
she studied surface design in London, developing
a passion for textiles and photography that would
inform the vision of her eponymous brand.

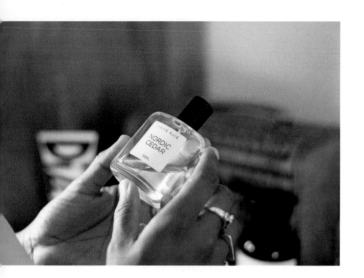

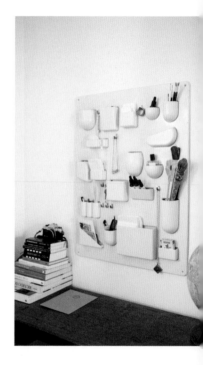

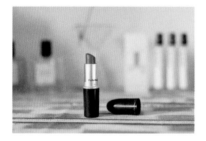

'I started sharing with people
where my inspirations came from.
Many sprung from my old family
photographs dating back through
the decades.'

After many years working in fashion retail, I did a surface design foundation degree as a mature student, mainly focusing on textiles and photography. Through my studies at the London College of Communication, I became interested in how I could implement scent in the visual work I was doing. I've always been drawn in by scent. Whether that's personal fragrance, home fragrance or beauty products, it's always been at the forefront of how I shop, so I've always wanted to draw people in with olfaction as well as visuals.

After my degree I took on a job that was not as creative as I had hoped it to be. During that time I was working front of house in an arts hub in Hackney. I had started experimenting with oils, and every time I made a fragrance I would bring it in and scent my work space. Throughout the years I spent there, I had daily conversations about fragrance as people would ask me about the scent in the reception. I didn't know at the time but these conversations ended up serving as my market research for what was to come.

I started sharing with people where my inspirations came from. Many sprung from my old family photographs dating back through the decades. At university I would put them on my mood boards and pair them with colour palettes in order for my tutors to follow my creative journey. People loved this multisensory experience; It's a powerful way of encountering picture, colour work and smell simultaneously, and this became my avenue into starting my brand.

I set up my company manufacturing from my kitchen table. Shortly after that I moved into a studio next to my house on the Isle of Dogs, and since then I've been producing from here, mainly on my own.

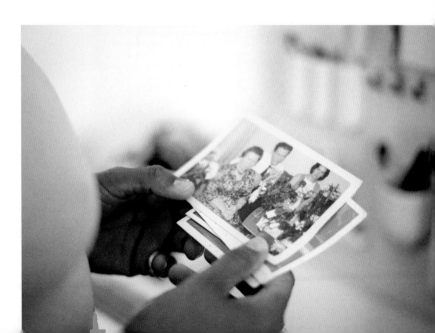

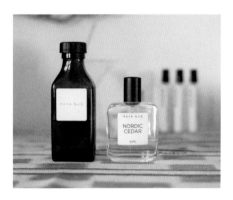

Rituals are important. I love exfoliating and I love moisturizing, and then I love applying scent. And I enjoy the ritual of a foot bath with salt and tea tree oil. I also have my candles, an incense burner and incense sticks that I light. I discovered a Cire Trudon limited edition called Philae, which is named after a temple. It's spiced pepper and cedar with papyrus, the kind of resinous and deep fragrance that I go for. They don't make it any more, so I have to scour for it and I have a stash of them now.

I stumbled across qigong by accident. It's a set of exercises that are connected to sounds. You tap your muscles and your joints and you make sounds and movement. It has a really calming effect, and it's a nice way to wake up your muscles. It's described as a mind, body, spirit practice that improves mental and physical health by integrating posture movement, breathing technique, sound and focused intent.

Growing up in Sweden I didn't feel like there was much of a beauty standard that catered for people of colour, the lack thereof pretty much became the norm. As I moved to London I felt like I fitted in more. Things like having better access to Afro haircare made a difference, it was pretty much non-existent back home at the time.

My beauty aesthetic is simple and minimalist. In terms of make-up, I tend to wear mascara and blusher, and if I run out of blusher I am happy to dab a bit of lipstick on my cheeks instead. I have a couple of friends who are make-up artists, and they know what colouring I am. They might give me a blusher or an eyebrow pen.

Fragrance can lift your mood. If you're feeling low and need a boost, put fragrance on and it will elevate you. Sometimes it's connected to nostalgia; it might make you think of somebody you love or have lost, and who you want to be close to again.

Citrus and florals are generally always uplifting. Bergamot, mandarin and grapefruit are three oils I like to use. Neroli also gives me a boost when I need one. I wear deeper, more narcotic florals too, ylang-ylang and orris I love to put in my skin oils. These are not your typical light, airy florals, they both have real depth and character to them.

I miss the Swedish lakes and being able to enjoy outdoor swimming, walking in the forests and that feeling only the midnight sun can give you; It's an ethereal light that lifts any mood. I'm probably the happiest around midsummer because of it, I try and time my visits back so I get a dose of it each year.

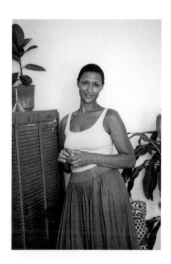

'Fragrance can lift your mood. If you're feeling low and need a boost, put fragrance on and it will elevate you. Sometimes it's connected to nostalgia; it might make you think of somebody you love or have lost, and who you want to be close to again.'

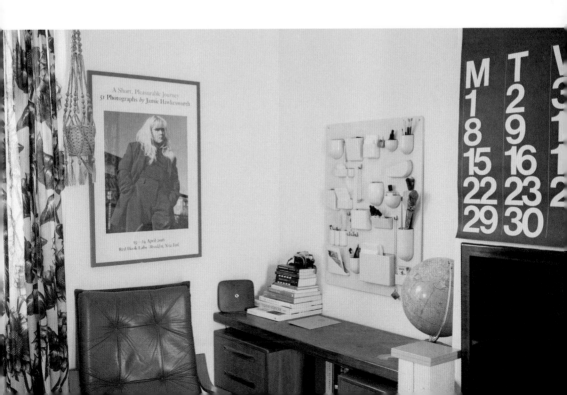

Ellen von Unwerth

FASHION PHOTOGRAPHER

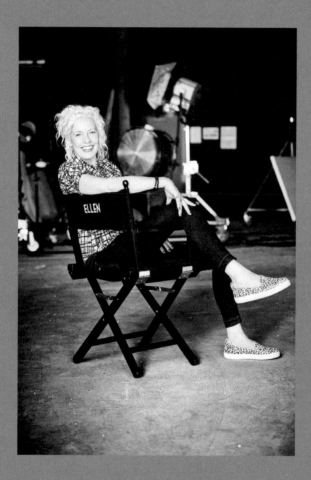

Ellen von Unwerth's celebratory fashion
photography is informed by her childhood
experiences and early career as a model.

I first became aware of style and beauty when I was chosen between other children from a line of orphans [by foster parents] at the age of three. I was also given little red boots, which I adored and which gave me the love for the colour red and a fetish for shoes.

My modelling days, which lasted for ten years, definitely shaped my approach to fashion and beauty photography. I was always frustrated as a model because I felt I was used more like a clothes hanger. But as a photographer I am more interested in the person I am photographing or the story I want to tell through the clothes, hair and make-up.

Physical beauty is something fascinating; it attracts you like a magnet. It can also fade into indifference, while something or somebody with charm and energy can be more emotional and have a longer lasting effect on you.

Beauty rituals? Love is all I need. But a nice lipstick always helps to make you feel glamorous and gives you the strength to conquer the world. And, of course, platinum hair for me!

I think diversity in the fashion industry is a big trend right now, which is great. It was needed for a long time. But we should also be aware that this trend was launched by marketing professionals who serve the cause of brands. I imagine that soon something else will come along.

'Love is all I need. But a nice lipstick always helps to make you feel glamorous and gives you the strength to conquer the world.'

For me it was always unquestionable that I would photograph people with different looks, genders or races. I also always like to be a bit provocative and push things forward. I remember when I shot two girls in fishnets kissing for *The Face* magazine. It was quite shocking for the readers and you wouldn't have seen it in *Vogue*, but today it is totally normal.

Nowadays, the casting system is shifting. The model agencies hold the girls back and wait for the 'big fish' jobs. But those jobs are increasingly rare and now we are swamped by lots of little ones. Magazines are slowly disappearing and everybody is looking at social media, with influencers taking the places of models and even actors. It is more about self-promotion and micro-celebrity today and people are more and more self-obsessed. On the other hand I am finding lots of interesting talents on Instagram, who I can connect and work with. Things are changing and you have to go with the flow – or not!

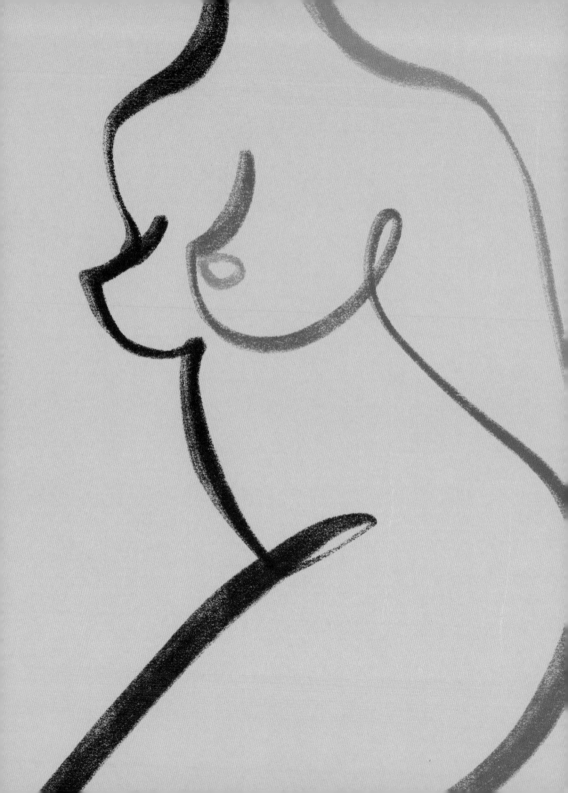

The Rituals:
Body

'I don't like to see beauty as torture,
or as a competition. I'm not interested at all
in being younger or thinner; I just want
to feel good in myself.' This statement
from Buly 1803 co-founder Victoire de
Taillac-Touhami really resonates with me.
It came during a conversation about her
love of bath-time rituals, and sums up the
approach of many of my interviewees to
self-care and feeling good.

Bathing rituals in particular stand out as an opportunity
to be at one with ourselves, even if we're surrounded by others.
From Korean spas to Moroccan hammams to Japanese onsens,
the combination of physical cleansing with mental offloading
is potent and sacred. 'In Japan, bathing is a part of life; when
you're tired, you take a bath,' says Ryoko Hori. 'In an onsen bath
it's also the social space where you communicate. You meet
people there and you just chat. Even though you're naked, it's
fine! You wash your body, but it's also like cleansing your
mental stress.'

Meanwhile, in a world where it can feel as though everything
is public, the bathroom is the one place where you can lock
the door and truly escape. A steaming tub with magnesium
flakes and therapeutic oils can even relieve chronic pain. The
feeling of warm water produces the bonding hormone oxytocin,
mimicking the feeling of comfort you get when you're with loved
ones. The higher the temperature, the better the endorphin rush
for easing pain and lifting your mood.

Adding oils and salts to a bath has many effects, from olfactory
to skin softening. Cleopatra, an icon for bathing rituals if ever

'If you respond to aromatherapy, try a lavender-infused body oil before bed to promote deep slumber.'

there was one, soaked in the soured milk of donkeys, while the French queen Marie Antoinette preferred pine nuts, linseed and sweet almond oil for fragrance and exfoliating. While there's big business in expensive bath potions, the humble magnesium-flake soak is equally effective at soothing aching muscles and boosting energy. Magnesium also helps the body to produce insulin, which regulates blood sugar and staves off mood swings.

While pre- and post-bath rituals may not sound as sexy as luxuriating in the tub, they have their own advantages. As I get older I've become evangelical about foot care, specifically filing my heels and soles once a week. Use a professional foot file on dry skin, starting at the top of the foot and working down to the heels. Not only will this prevent hard skin and corns from building up, it's also extremely satisfying and – dare I say it – almost meditative.

Dry body brushing is an equally invigorating pre-bath (or shower) ritual. Originating in the Ayurvedic practice of *garshana* (from the Sanskrit 'friction by rubbing'), the process stimulates a sluggish lymphatic system, strengthens immunity and softens the overall tone of the skin. Using a firm bristle brush, apply sweeping strokes from feet to knees, from knees to hips, over the bum and torso, and from hands to shoulders. Repeat a few times for each section, always in the direction of the heart.

After the bath or shower, while the skin is still warm, is the best time to massage in nourishing body creams, oils and balms. 'I use the body balm by 79 Lux, or I mix it up by using baobab oil, moringa oil and coconut oil, with organic shea butter that I buy in bulk from the north of Ghana,' says the actor Marie Humbert. The age-management consultant and 79 Lux skincare founder Karen Cummings-Palmer reinforces the virtues of her balm. 'The human touch is wonderful therapy,' she says. 'It releases the feel-good hormones dopamine and serotonin, increasing our sense of happiness and wellbeing. The simple act of self-massage using a good-quality balm or oil will also yield benefits.' Her balm was formulated to treat her own eczema-prone skin, and contains rose quartz for its self-soothing and circulation boosting properties.

If you respond to aromatherapy, try a lavender-infused body oil before bed to promote deep slumber. Cup your hands and inhale from your palms after massaging it into your skin. Both Votary Night Oil and the cult Dr Hauschka Moor Lavender Calming Body Oil deliver a soporific knockout.

The key to overall body maintenance at any age is regular gentle movement. Holistic practices including qigong, yoga and the Feldenkrais Method integrate posture movement with breathing techniques and focused intent. For anyone who spends hours folded over a computer keyboard or phone screen, frequent simple stretches may be enough to unknot stiff limbs and muscles. My Feldenkrais tip is to hold your smartphone at eye level instead of in the hunchback 'tech neck' position. You can fold the other arm across your body so that your fist serves as an elbow rest. Cummings-Palmer encourages standing up when taking calls, and pulling the tummy to the spine and rolling the shoulders back when sitting at a desk. Even better? Get (far, far) away from the desk at any opportunity.

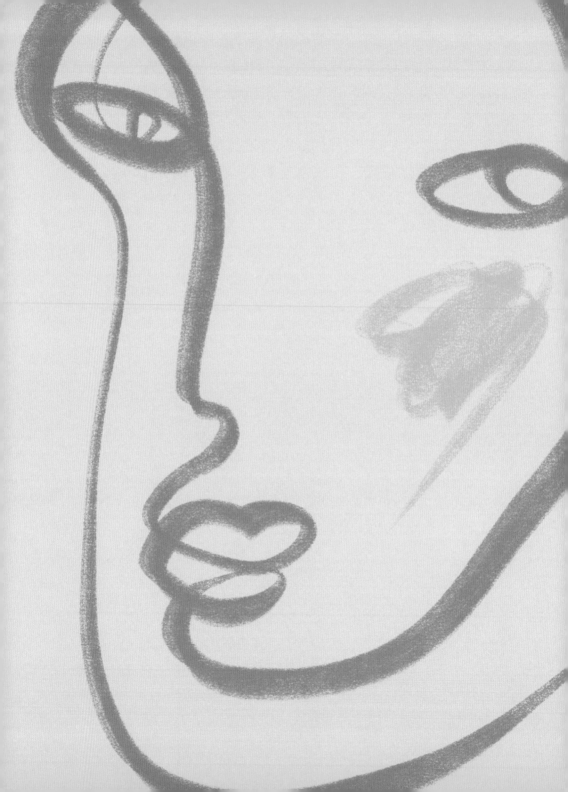

The Beauty Cabinet

Inside the ritualist's beauty cabinet lies a capsule
edit of make-up, skincare and holistic tools.
Whether you prefer plant-based 'clean' beauty
or lab-grown hi-tech skincare, here's what to buy,
how to use it and where it fits into your routine.
Remember, for products to be effective,
follow a logical order, allow them time to work
and address problem skin one concern at a time.

Toothpaste

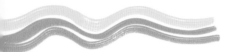

Here's the thing about oral care: it just isn't sexy. But it's hugely important to our overall physical health and how we feel about ourselves.

The study of the human microbiome can be traced back to 1683, when a self-taught scientist, Antonie van Leeuwenhoek, discovered the bacteria in his dental plaque. Centuries later we now know that mouth microbes give a window into the inner workings of our bodies, and that minimizing the number of bacteria in our mouths can help to prevent certain health conditions.

Chiming with this knowledge of the importance of oral health is a new generation of wellness-focused oral-care products. At the forefront of the movement are the sensorial toothpastes from Lebon and Buly 1803 – both French companies, of course! Their delicious – and chicly packaged – pastes use natural ingredients and gourmet flavours such as orange blossom, rose and mint to make the humdrum ritual a pleasure, not a chore. Equally elegant for the most inelegant of practices are the upscale dental flosses that aim to shift the stubborn dental debris clinging to our molars. Try Buly's apple-scented beeswax-coated floss or the mango-flavoured variety from Cocofloss to elevate your flossing regime.

Another oral hygiene ritual that is gaining surprising traction is the Ayurvedic practice of oil pulling. This holistic (and affordable) process of removing bacteria by swishing sesame or coconut oil around your mouth is also considered somewhat meditative. Not only have studies shown that it can help to reduce harmful bacteria, but anecdotal evidence also suggests that it can whiten teeth without the need for bleaching agents.

Continuing the Ayurvedic influence, tongue scraping is another satisfying ritual for the oral-obsessed. Consider a couple of minutes of tongue scraping to energize you during a mid-afternoon slump, instead of a caffeine hit. Buly's Victoire de Taillac-Touhami is a fan: '[It's] genius when you don't feel great. You really have the feeling that you're very clean after cleaning your tongue.'

WHERE TO SHOP:

Aēsop, Buly 1803, Cocofloss, Keeko, Lebon, Twice

Cleanser

Who would have thought that the tedium of washing your face would be reinvented as a near-spiritual feel-good exercise? But massaging oils, balms or creams into the skin has become a pleasant daily ritual for millions of people.

Oils are a special type of solvent because they are lipophilic, meaning they attract and break down other oils, including those in make-up and the sebum in our skin. The best non-pore-clogging oil cleansers are those formulated with added emulsifiers. They liquefy into a milk before being rinsed off. The Japanese do it best in this case, with Shu Uemura, DHC and even Muji offering plant-based oils that clean and nourish the skin.

Melting solid balms and milky jelly cleansers have a similar pleasurable tactility. Glossier Milky Jelly Cleanser, Beauty Pie Japanfusion Pure Transforming Cleanser and CeraVe Hydrating Cleanser give a clean result without stripping the skin and leaving it feeling tight, as do the rinse-off balms by Clinique, Pixi and the Body Shop.

WHERE TO SHOP:

**Beauty Pie, Bobbi Brown, Clinique, DHC,
Epara, Glossier, Muji, Pixi, Shu Uemura, Typology**

Serum

Where to start with serums? These are the little bottles of active potions designed to penetrate the skin most deeply. You apply them straight on to your skin (before moisturizer, facial oil or SPF) to target specific concerns, from dullness, acne or scarring to sun damage. They can also be added to moisturizer to boost its benefits.

While some serums focus on one hero active ingredient, others combine a few in a potent cocktail. Research your chosen serum and proceed slowly; it's best to start with smaller concentrations of active ingredients. And don't be greedy. 'For things to be effective you have to commit to them. Give them time; don't layer too many things,' cautions the wellness entrepreneur Ariana Mouyiaris. 'You're not going to wear five serums; they're just going to clog your pores.'

Of the myriad serums available, a few are universally lauded. 'Acid toning' serums are liquid exfoliators that resurface the skin, leaving it smoother and brighter, such as Tata Harper Resurfacing Serum, a combination of plant-based acids. Remember always to follow acid toner serums with sun protection, however. Vitamin C is the antioxidant serum that will boost overall radiance, targeting dullness, dark spots and hyper-pigmentation. Dr Dennis Gross, Drunk Elephant and Kiehl's are all excellent. Niacinamide is the technical name for vitamin B3 serum that soothes, heals and helps to make more collagen. Medik8 Clarity Peptides is the high-end choice, while The Ordinary's Niacinamide 10% + Zinc 1% is the well-loved budget option that reduces bacteria and calms the skin.

WHERE TO SHOP:

**Disciple Typology, Dr Dennis Gross,
Drunk Elephant, Elequra, Kiehl's, Medik8,
Nairian, The Ordinary, Tata Harper**

Moisturizer

A basic moisturizer should contain a humectant (such as glycerine) to attract water to the skin, emollient oils to trap the water, plus barrier-boosting ingredients (such as ceramides and niacinamide) to strengthen the microbiome. Over and above that, the new generation of multitasking moisturizers are supercharged with active ingredients, which makes them more expensive, but will help streamline your routine. Just be careful not to overdose accidentally by adding a serum that duplicates the actions.

The gel-cream moisturizers are particularly appealing. Originating in South Korea – the epicentre of all things future-facing – they marry a weightless feeling on the face with skin-repairing ingredients. Glow Recipe Watermelon Glow Pink Juice is great for those who suffer from oily skin, with its botanical extracts and moisture-sealing hyaluronic acid. Clinique Moisture Surge is another bouncy gel that uses aloe water, caffeine and hyaluronic acid to attract and lock in moisture.

For a more traditional cream texture, I like Beauty Pie Japanfusion Urban Air Purifying Day Moisturizer, which contains Japanese active ingredients to calm and purify the skin, while Chanel Hydra Beauty Camellia Water Cream is wonderfully weightless and imparts a subtle light-reflective radiance. For the summer, La Mer The Radiant Skintint moisturizes, fights damage caused by pollution and gives a sun-kissed gleam.

While there's an ongoing war between so-called 'clean beauty' and 'chemical' skincare, I have time for both. Tata Harper is one of the most revered plant-based brands, a favourite with the boutique owner Linda V. Wright (page 64), who appreciates the brand's eco philosophy and its benefits for her mature skin.

Ultimately, it's important to realize that face creams are cosmetics, and the effects last only for the duration that you're using the product. When you stop using it, your skin will revert to the usual ageing process. So enjoy using the products, but do also accept that you can't 'reverse time'.

WHERE TO SHOP:

Beauty Pie, Chanel, Clinique, Glow Recipe, La Mer, Tata Harper

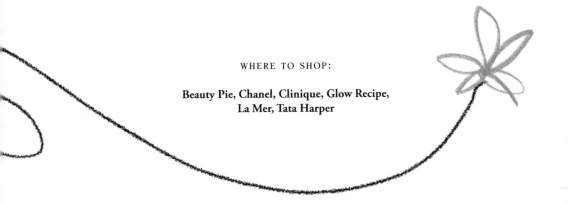

Facial Oil

Facial oils are, unsurprisingly, extremely popular among ritualists. Because they don't contain water, they don't need preservatives, so they satisfy the beauty minimalists who like as few ingredients as possible in their products.

Which oils to choose, then? While the main function is to trap moisture, facial oils also boast a wealth of skincare advantages. For general skin strengthening, repair and calming, look for prickly-pear seed, rosehip, rose and jasmine oils. Oily skins respond to lightweight oils, including ylang-ylang, jojoba and squalane. If you have dry skin, look for an oil that is rich in omega and fatty acids – marula oil is an excellent all-rounder.

If you want an oil that works for everything, including shaving, cleansing and beard grooming, try Everyday Oil. This super-oil comes in two varieties; a plain, non-scented version containing coconut, olive, argan, jojoba and castor oils, as well as the signature blend, Mainstay, with Palo Santo, lavender, geranium and clary sage essential oils. Remember that essential oils can irritate sensitive skin, so pick the version of Everyday Oil that suits your skin's needs.

To apply facial oil, simply pour a few drops into your palm, press your hands together 'top to toe' and swipe. Then gently press them to your face. Alternatively, add a few drops to boost your moisturizer. You can also use face oil to lubricate the skin for facial massage. The action of manipulating the skin and facial muscles with this viscous, almost blood-like substance is pleasantly life-affirming.

WHERE TO SHOP:

**Buly 1803, Drunk Elephant, Everyday Oil,
The Ordinary, Typology, Uma**

Facial Tool

Facial massage using the fingertips, palms and knuckles has proven stress-busting benefits. But better still are the moves carried out using a tool and targeting specific areas.

Enter the Gua Sha, a rose quartz or jade tool and ritual stemming from traditional Chinese medicine that helps to improve blood circulation, lymphatic drainage and skin elasticity. You scrape the angled, smooth-edged stone along the contours of the face using regular upward-and-outward movements to lift the internal connective tissue. To help the Gua Sha glide more easily, use a facial oil. As an added incentive, the technique will help the oil penetrate the skin.

Gua Sha can also be used on the scalp and body, but consistency is crucial. Two to three minutes a day will result in long-term changes to the skin structure, while releasing underlying tension.

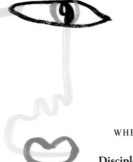

WHERE TO SHOP:

Disciple, Hayo'u, Odacité

Sun Protection

One of the reasons 'anti-ageing' products are so popular is that people of my generation spent way too much time smoking while sizzling in the sun in the 1980s. But while we're well versed in skin repair, sun protection is still something of a minefield. Quite simply, the best way to stop your skin from being damaged by the sun is to avoid going out in it. The sun is most brutal between 11 am and 3 pm, so that's the time to stay in the shade under a giant hat, sunglasses and a supersize shirt.

Failing that, load up on UVA and UVB protection. UVA protects against skin ageing, while UVB protects against skin cancer, so we need both. There are two types of formula to choose from. 'Physical' sunscreen reflects UV radiation using titanium dioxide and zinc oxide, but its thick, white consistency can be hard to blend. Dermalogica's Invisible Physical Defense SPF30 is a good solution.

Meanwhile, 'chemical' sunscreen absorbs UV radiation and is usually lighter and easier to blend.

For example, Glossier's Invisible Shield has a water-gel formula that is friendly to sensitive skin, while the excellent La Roche-Posay Anthelios Ultra-Light Invisible Fluid Sun Cream comes in a lightweight fluid and handy mini size.

Caution: While moisturizer with added SPF may protect against small amounts of sun exposure (such as walking to the car), the British Association of Dermatologists advises using a dedicated sunscreen for longer exposure. And, despite the persistent misconception, dark skin also needs protection. '[Such skin] may be slow to wrinkle, but the sun will cause collagen to break down, increased pigmentation and uneven skin tone,' cautions the age-management consultant Karen Cummings-Palmer. Both the organic SPF30 chemical sunscreen by the Danish brand Ecooking and Murad City Skin Age Defense Broad Spectrum SPF50 (with vitamin C and a matte finish) are endorsed by the Black Skin Directory.

WHERE TO SHOP:

Dermalogica, Ecooking, Glossier, Kiehl's, Murad, La Roche-Posay, Shiseido

Foundation and Concealer

The beauty equivalent of a pair of jeans, foundation is utterly personal and depends on many factors. You feel as though you've won the lottery when you finally find 'your' shade and formulation. I still remember my first, Prescriptives Virtual Skin in Real Beige yellow/orange. It really was like real skin.

The job of foundation is to even out skin tone, not cover up the skin completely. Thankfully, today's formulations combine pigment with skincare benefits, giving them the most natural-looking finish yet. Gucci Westman (page 96) launched her Westman Atelier Vital Skin foundation to calm and minimize the redness caused by her rosacea. It contains antioxidants and active ingredients, including squalane to restore suppleness and camellia-seed oil to protect the skin from environmental pollutants.

Bobbi Brown has always been great for foundation, with a broad spectrum of shades and textures for every skin tone. The foundation stick is a classic for on-the-go touch-ups, and its slightly dry formula makes it good for mattifying shine-prone skin. MAC, NARS and Estée Lauder also offer extensive shade ranges. To compare shades online, Findation.com is a clever tool.

Fenty Beauty changed the game for everyone when it launched with 50 shades in 2017. Its Pro Filt'r Soft Matte Longwear Foundation contains 'climate-adaptive' technology that makes it resistant to sweat and humidity. The hi-tech Japanese brands are also leaders in innovative formulations for humid environments. Shiseido Synchro Skin Self-Refreshing foundation uses smart technology to repel sweat and oil, while Koh Gen Do Aqua Foundation is recommended by the model Taira (page 112) for its luminous but shine-busting powers. For the ultimate 'no make-up' foundation, Armani Beauty's Luminous Silk foundation is a long-standing favourite thanks to its lightweight, oil-free formula.

On the concealer front, NARS Radiant Creamy Concealer is the insiders' choice for under eyes, while Glossier Stretch Concealer is a rare formulation that works equally well on dark shadows, redness and spots.

WHERE TO SHOP:

Armani Beauty, Bobbi Brown, Burberry, Estée Lauder, Fenty Beauty, Glossier, Koh Gen Do, MAC, NARS, Shiseido, Westman Atelier

Highlighter

For a few years there was a trend for 'lit' cheekbones that you could see from the moon. This isn't that. Highlighters should be applied sparingly, to add just a suggestion of luminosity to the high points of the face. The effect should emulate the gentle, ethereal glow of a Renaissance portrait. The make-up artist Gucci Westman (page 96) is famed for achieving this dimensional look by using highlighter before *and* after foundation. The first application goes on the tops of the cheekbones, in the corners of the eyes and above the Cupid's bow. After foundation, her Westman Atelier Super Loaded Tinted Highlight goes on the cheekbones and across the eyelids. 'The layering of different highlighters is what creates luminous, dewy skin,' she says.

If that sounds too labour-intensive, there's a simplified version. Use a sheer, balm-like stick, such as Glossier Haloscope or Chanel Baume Essentiel Multi-use Glow Stick just on the tops of the cheekbones and eyelids. The make-up artist Shinobu Abe uses the bronze version on male and female clients to gently warm up the complexion. MAC Strobe Cream and RMS Beauty Luminizer pots are also firm favourites, while Glossier Futuredew is an all-over water-in-oil serum that imparts a Michelangelo-worthy radiance. (Unlike Michelangelo, use fingers rather than brushes for speedy application.)

Caution: On dark skin, too-light highlighter will look ashy, while yellow-gold can look unnatural, so aim for a bronze tint such as Pat McGrath Labs Skin Fetish Highlighter and Balm Duo.

WHERE TO SHOP:

**Chanel, Glossier, Kevyn Aucoin, MAC,
Pat McGrath Labs, RMS, Westman Atelier**

Blusher

Blusher is my go-to, wake-me-up product for when I'm looking or feeling lacklustre. As we age, we lose colour in our cheeks and lips, not to mention the pigment in our hair, all of which can make us look washed out.

I gravitate towards cream blushes that can be applied quickly with the fingers. Chanel Rouge Coco Lip Blush has a light gel texture, and Bobbi Brown Pot Rouge is great for a deeper pay-off. I like to apply mine below the apples of the cheeks, and a little across the bridge of the nose. If it's a warmer, terracotta tone, I dab it on the eyelids as well.

For a polished finish, switch cream blusher for powder and apply it with a brush. Powder also has more staying power than cream, especially on oily skin. NARS blushers are finely milled and come in a good spectrum of shades.

Don't forget your undertone. Dark skins suit plum shades, olive and yellow undertones suit peach, and pink undertones look good in rose or berry.

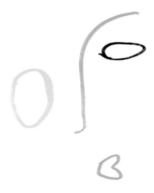

WHERE TO SHOP:

Bobbi Brown, Chanel, Glossier, Kevyn Aucoin, Kjaer Weis, Kosas, NARS

Bronzer

In summer, when I want to go barefaced but still like some added oomph, I turn to bronzer. This isn't about replicating a tan (more on that below), but rather about enlivening the complexion enough to suggest health and vitality. The irony of darker-than-natural skin is that it's a sign not of health but of burning. So perhaps what we're trying to achieve is the *feeling* of being outdoors in the sun, rather than the reality.

I don't like putting in much effort, which is why I like cream bronzer. A solid cream, such as Chanel Healthy Glow Bronzing Cream, can be blended easily into the hairline, under the jaw and across the nose and high points of the cheeks using a kabuki brush. Milk Makeup's vegan-friendly Matte Bronzer stick is equally malleable and buildable.

A little blusher on cheeks and sheer lip gloss complete the summer-in-the-Balearics look. If cream isn't your preferred texture, or if you have oily skin, go for a powder bronzer, but apply sparingly. Guerlain Terracotta The Bronzing Powder, Chanel Les Beiges Healthy Glow Sheer Powder and Tom Ford Soleil Glow Bronzer are the matte formulations to look for.

If you want to replicate a tan in the easiest, most natural-looking way, consider self-tanning drops. Add three drops to your serum or moisturizer, blend well into the skin – quickly! – and watch the colour develop gradually over a couple of days. Dr Sebagh and Tan-Luxe are the ones I recommend.

WHERE TO SHOP:

**Chanel, Guerlain, Dr Sebagh, Milk Makeup,
Tan-Luxe, Tom Ford**

Eyeshadow

When it comes to easy-to-use eyeshadows, I'm a big fan of cream-to-powder formulations. You can apply them with the fingertips to warm up the product and help it blend effortlessly.

If you're lazy or time-poor, or just prefer an understated look, use classic neutrals. Taupes and bone shadows are good on their own for basic grooming, or as a base underneath darker shades. Khaki and rich browns suit everyone, and I love a dark aubergine as an unusual neutral.

Chanel's Ombre Première and Chantecaille's Mermaid Eye Mattes are my favourite pot shadows.

Laura Mercier's Caviar Stick Eye Colour and Bobbi Brown's Long-wear Cream Shadow Stick are the stick equivalents: super-malleable to apply and blend into the lash line.

For almost-nothingy make-up, I love a balm or eye gloss. MAKE Dew Pot is a perfect barely there lid balm that just adds a little definition, while Kevyn Aucoin's The Exotique Diamond Eye Gloss gives a wet-look effect on the lids, and works well on its own or over another colour.

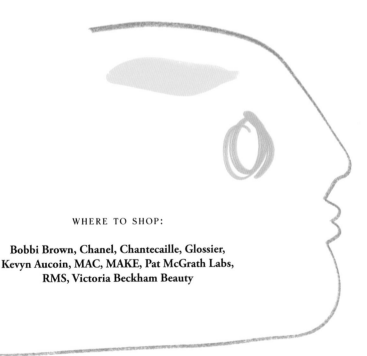

WHERE TO SHOP:

Bobbi Brown, Chanel, Chantecaille, Glossier, Kevyn Aucoin, MAC, MAKE, Pat McGrath Labs, RMS, Victoria Beckham Beauty

Brow Gel

Good brows can make a great difference to the face. They draw attention to the eyes and accentuate emotional expression. I take my brow cues from boys; I prefer them as straight as possible and untampered-with, but tidy. Too tweezed or waxed and they can look severe, particularly if you have strong features. The more you let them grow and just keep them groomed, the easier the upkeep.

I like sharp tweezers for keeping strays at bay between the brows, and just a bit of brow gel to keep the hairs in place. Browcote or MAC Brow Set are my clear gels of choice, and Glossier Boy Brow is good if you need a slight tint. Its tiny brush means it's hard to over-apply. Stroke the brows upwards with a comb, then apply the gel sparingly.

If brow hairs are excessively long, just comb them upwards and snip the overhang with sharp nail scissors. If brows are sparse, cold-pressed castor oil can help with growth. The wellness coach Isa-Welly Locoh-Donou (page 40) and Cosmic Cosmic founder Ariana Mouyiaris (page 48) both apply it fastidiously. (It works on lashes, too.)

Brows lose pigment with age, and this can make the complexion look washed out. To increase the contrast, consider tinted gel, or a hard, waxy pencil if you prefer. Boy de Chanel and Tom Ford are recommended for their sharp, angled nibs. Choose a shade lighter than your natural colour and use feathery strokes to mimic each hair. A good tip is to steady your elbow on a firm surface and hold the pencil nearer the end to give you a looser wrist action. Other than these tiny hair flicks, avoid the temptation to draw an extended line across the brow.

WHERE TO SHOP:

Browcote, Chanel, Glossier, MAC, Tom Ford

Mascara

Not everyone wants super-long, super-thick, OTT eyelashes. For some people, a little definition is better than a full Bambi flutter. I default to Clinique and Lancôme for soft, natural-looking mascara that won't transfer to the lower lids. In fact, I just apply it to the top lashes, slowly lifting the brush up and outwards to elongate the lash line. Clear mascara is another option; it has a subtle effect that's good for dark lashes. Maybelline Great Lash Washable Mascara in Clear does the job at an affordable price.

If you do want something a little more substantial, Dior's Diorshow mascara gives length and definition without chunkiness. And for those with poker-straight lashes who need help cultivating curl, DHC Mascara Perfect Pro Double Protection is a Japanese 'tubing' mascara with a thin brush that coats each lash precisely and without clumping.

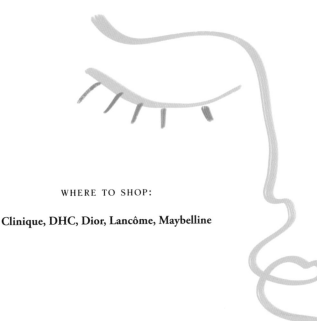

WHERE TO SHOP:

Clinique, DHC, Dior, Lancôme, Maybelline

Lipstick

Make-up trends come and go, but let's all agree, you can't beat a minimalist face adorned with nothing but a true red lip. OK, perhaps also some concealer and mascara and a fingertip of sheer highlighter, but the mouth is where the eye needs to go.

I love the casual look of a stain. According to the make-up artist Shinobu Abe, the key is first to apply a waxy lip balm ('Carmex is fine, not too much'), then to dab the lipstick straight from the bullet using a clean finger. Blot the excess with a tissue and use your fingers to tidy the edge. 'Much less wasteful than using a cotton bud!' says Abe.

For a non-drying stain, you need an emollient lipstick such as the Chanel Rouge Coco Stylo stick, which is well pigmented yet balmy. Matte formulations are a little more intense and have more staying power. Liquid lip inks are wonderful (I like Revlon Ultra HD Matte Lip Mousse and Armani Beauty Lip Magnet), but MAC lipsticks are the undisputed red lipstick leaders, with seven tubes of Ruby Woo sold every minute. I sometimes put a clear lip gloss on top and blot that, too.

Growing eco concerns have given us some new waste-free packaging concepts, and particularly worth mentioning are the refillable luxury lipsticks by La Bouche Rouge, Hermès and Charlotte Tilbury. La Bouche Rouge specializes in serum-infused reds of every description, but also does some classic rose-beiges, pinks and balms. (My 83-year-old mum is a fan.) The casing of the lipstick is not only refillable, but also free of microplastics, with the aim of keeping harmful plastic waste out of the world's oceans. Vegan beauty is another major consumer concern. Milk Makeup, whose cruelty-free lipsticks are a firm favourite of the artist and jeweller Arpana Rayamajhi (page 92), makes its demi-matte reds and pinks with shea butter, coconut oil and grapeseed oil.

Finally, a word on the basics. For a really simple and moisturizing lip balm with a hint of a tint, Bobbi Brown Extra Lip Tint in any of its lip-mimicking shades is an excellent all-dayer.

WHERE TO SHOP:

**Armani Beauty, Bobbi Brown,
La Bouche Rouge, Chanel, Charlotte Tilbury,
Hermès, MAC, Milk Makeup, Revlon**

Fragrance

For evoking calm, focus and positivity, nature-inspired fragrances tend to be universally loved. This is hardly surprising, since they inevitably trigger memories of childhood holidays and outdoorsy exploits. In particular, juicy citruses and herbaceous colognes are easy to wear and energizing for the spirit, a reminder of the days when colognes were used as a medicinal pick-me-up.

Perfumer H Orange Leaf eau de parfum is a perennial favourite of mine, as is any Hermès cologne. Santa Maria Novella colognes transport me to its incredible pharmacy in Florence, where Dominican monks first concocted herbal remedies in the thirteenth century. And the cool musk-meets-lavender notes of Chanel's Jersey eau de parfum instantly take me back to family holidays in the heat and dust of 1980s Bombay.

Dry body oils are another way to wear scent, while also nourishing the skin. Nuxe's cult Huile Prodigieuse and NARS Monoï Body Glow are just two that can conjure faraway beaches from the comfort of a suburban sofa.

Don't turn your nose up at high-street fragrances. I have a well-loved & Other Stories Moroccan Tea eau de toilette that's long discontinued but still restores my equilibrium with a single spritz.

While the perfume industry has historically thrived on old-school glamour codes, changes are afoot in the age of responsibility and transparency. Indie perfumers such as Maya Njie and Floral Street offer minimal packaging, while Sana Jardin's circular business model enables the women in its supply chain to become micro-entrepreneurs by upcycling waste from its perfume production.

Recognizing this shift, the luxury perfumer Acqua di Parma recently produced Colonia Futura, its first cologne made from 99 per cent natural ingredients. And the blockchain platform Provenance helps online retailers share brands' eco and ethical credentials with customers through its rigorous traceability system.

WHERE TO SHOP:

& Other Stories, Acqua di Parma, Buly 1803, Chanel, Floral Street, Hermès, Maya Njie, Perfumer H, Sana Jardin, Santa Maria Novella

Morning and Evening Rituals

Morning Ritual

It's important to know *what* to do *when* in your daily routine to maximize the benefits. For each skincare product to be effective, you must follow a logical line-up. In the case of strong active ingredients, err on the side of caution and address one skincare concern at a time, rather than loading on lots of aggressive lotions. Skincare has become a fashion pastime, but peer pressure and the 'must-have' culture are not the best way to care for your skin.

For daytime, the simplest running order goes: cleanser, toner, serum, moisturizer, facial oil, SPF. For evening, you can leave out the SPF and maybe add some of the stronger acid serums. However, if you have problem skin, it's advisable to consult a doctor or dermatologist before trying harsh products.

ORAL CARE
Brush your teeth as soon as you get up. Avoid brushing for at least 30 minutes after eating anything acidic.

CLEANSER
Removes surface dirt, sweat and oil and prepares the skin to receive active products.

TONER OR FACIAL MIST (OPTIONAL)
Removes the last traces of cleanser and refreshes the skin.

HYDRATING SERUM
Keeps the skin plumped while protecting it from dryness and free radicals.

MOISTURIZER
Use a moisturizer with a humectant to pull in water from the air, and an emollient to counter the taut feeling caused by drying soaps and cleansers.

FACIAL OIL (OPTIONAL)
If you like extra hydration or have dry skin. If you have oily skin, skip this step or save it for night-time.

SPF
Sun protection always goes last. Think of it as a direct physical shield against sun damage.

COFFEE, MEDITATION, YOGA, QIQONG, RUNNING, BODY BRUSHING …
Whatever you need to set yourself up for the rest of the day.

Evening Ritual

UNWIND
Decompress with some gentle yoga, meditation, an aromatherapy bath or a facial massage. At the very least, turn off messaging apps for an hour before bed.

DOUBLE-CLEANSE
If you wear make-up, double-cleanse at night: once with an oily or balmy cleanser to break down make-up and SPF, and again with a mild foaming cleanser to clean the skin itself.

EXFOLIATING/ACID TONER
(OPTIONAL, ONCE OR TWICE A WEEK)
Exfoliates and brightens the skin, clears breakouts and fades pigmentation. Removing the surface cells makes the skin underneath susceptible to sun damage, so save this step for the evening.

SERUM
Add your night-time repair ingredients. (If you're using an exfoliating toner, check that you're not duplicating any active ingredients.)

MOISTURIZER
Use your regular moisturizer, or consider a heavier night cream if you have dry skin.

FACIAL OIL
Apply with facial massage using your fingers or a tool such as a Gua Sha stone. Use an aromatherapy oil (unless you're sensitive) for its heightened relaxation powers.

ORAL CARE
Leave this until last. Wait an hour after eating to brush your teeth. Start with mouthwash, then floss, then brush for two minutes. Spit out the toothpaste but don't rinse; it will continue working in your mouth while you sleep. If you're interested in oil pulling, do it before your usual oral-care routine; just make sure you haven't eaten for at least two hours before.

GET A GOOD NIGHT'S SLEEP
If you have trouble sleeping, start dimming the lights a couple of hours before bed, and limit mental stimulation. Try a meditation app such as Calm or an aromatherapy pillow spray to encourage deep relaxation.

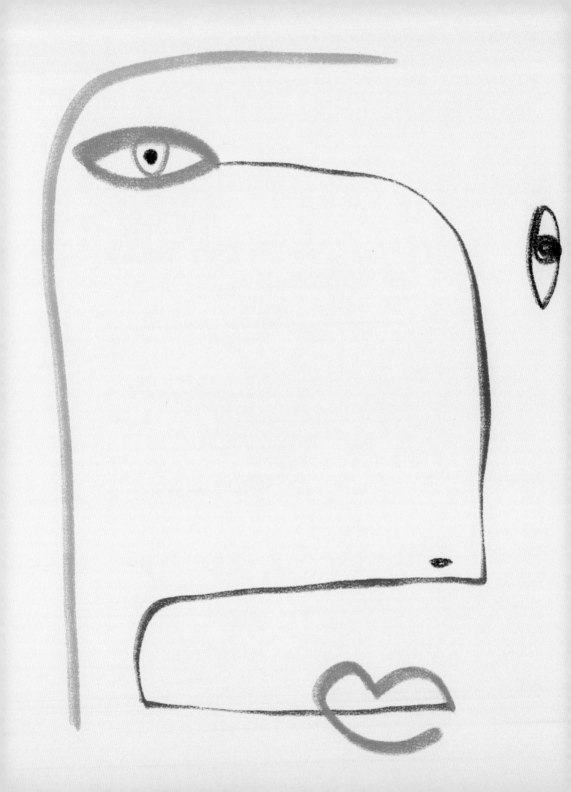

The B-List

From wellness destinations to retail playgrounds,
skincare brands to art museums, consult this list of
resources for expert beauty recommendations.

Wellbeing

Bathhouse
103 North 10th Street,
Brooklyn, NY 11249
abathhouse.com

-

This modern-day spa in a converted factory in Williamsburg offers Thai massages, hammam scrubs and a flotation tank.

Black Isle Bakery
Weinbergsweg 23, 10119 Berlin
blackislebakery.com

-

Ruth Barry's Berlin bakery serves artisan breads and treats overlooked by a Pieter Vermeersch art installation.

Celsious
115 North 7th Street,
Brooklyn, NY 11249
celsious.com

-

Theresa and Corinna Williams's reinvented laundrette for the eco era.

Cosmic Cosmic (opening 2022)
28 Gransden Avenue, Ground Floor,
London E8 3QA
cosmiccosmic.co

-

Ariana Mouyiaris's modern healing space brings the traditional retreat to city living.

Disciple
disciplelondon.com

-

Skin- and mind-calming oils, mists and serums from the psychotherapist Charlotte Ferguson.

Herboristerie
11 rue des Petits-Champs, 75001 Paris
herboristerie.com

-

Buly 1803 co-founder Victoire de Taillac-Touhami heads to this Palais Royal herb store for all her plant and oil wellbeing needs.

Susanne Kaufmann Spa
Hotel Post Bezau, Brugg 35
6870 Bezau
susannekaufmann.com

-

The wellness entrepreneur's spa combines restorative Eastern and Western practices using her signature plant-based skin and body care products

Keeko
keekooil.com

-

Elevated oral care inspired by Ayurvedic practices. Pick up your tongue scraper and oil-pulling tips here.

Senses
Friedelstraße 11, 12047 Berlin
ryoko-berlin.com

-

Ryoko Hori's massage spa, smell ritual space and meditation workshops combine with an artisan store to elevate the senses.

Sun Potion
sunpotion.com

-

The DJ and producer Honey Dijon's go-to site for shea butter, adaptogenic supplement powders and all things herbal.

Taza
tazaayurveda.com

-

Authentic Ayurvedic oils and supplements for the modern age.

Terahaku
terahaku.jp

-

For the ultimate in spiritual solace, stay in one of Japan's Buddhist 'temple stay' monasteries for tourists, known as shukubo. Terahaku is considered the Airbnb of temple accommodation.

Toraya
10 rue Saint Florentin, 75001 Paris
toraya-group.co.jp/toraya-paris

-

Linda V. Wright's favourite Japanese tea salon in Paris. Stop by for an energizing matcha tea or refreshing kakigori shaved ice with green tea and red bean paste.

Cultural Destinations

Blue Mountain School
9 Chance Street,
London E2 7JB
bluemountain.school
-

*Shoreditch's unique multi-disciplinary
space combining fashion, dining, music,
design, art and fragrance. Try the rooftop
tea experience for some respite from the
city*

The Feuerle Collection
Hallesches Ufer 70, 10963 Berlin
thefeuerlecollection.org
-

*Recommended by the massage therapist
Ryoko Hori, this private collection of
contemporary art and antiques is her
escape from the outside world.*

David Hill Gallery
345 Ladbroke Grove,
London W10 6HA
davidhillgallery.net
-

*Discover under-represented portrait and
reportage photography from Hill's roster
of international talent*

Gallery 1957
Kempinski Hotel
Gold Coast City & Galleria Mall,
PMB 66 – Ministries,
Gamel Abdul Nasser Avenue,
Ridge – Accra
gallery1957.com
-

*The actor and art advocate Marie
Humbert works with this gallery in
Accra to spot and promote the rising art
stars of West Africa.*

The Makeup Museum
94 Gansevoort Street,
New York, NY 10014
makeupmuseum.com
-

*Displaying iconic artefacts, cultural
ephemera and beauty products to
nostalgic make-up geeks and history
buffs.*

Mariane Ibrahim Gallery
437 N. Paulina Street
Chicago, IL 60622
marianeibrahim.com
-

*This Chicago gallerist is on a mission to
promote African artists, championing
up-and-coming talent from across the
continent*

Georgia O'Keeffe Museum
217 Johnson Street,
Santa Fe, NM 87501
okeeffemuseum.org
-

*The New Mexican museum is the
guardian of O'Keeffe's nature-inspired
work, while also maintaining the artist's
two homes and studios, a research centre,
library, plus a variety of related art
collections.*

Victoria and Albert Museum
Cromwell Road,
London SW7 2RL
vam.ac.uk
-

*Visit London's revered art and design
destination for its fashion exhibitions,
photography collection and Arts and
Crafts cafe.*

Perfumers and Scent

Acqua di Parma
acquadiparma.com
-
Transport yourself to the Italian coast with these classic colognes, creams and hair products.

Byredo
byredo.com
-
The Byredo empire encompasses leather goods, make-up, candles and accessories, but it all starts with founder Ben Gorham's innovative, emotion-led perfumes.

Cire Trudon
trudon.com
-
The oldest candlemaker in the world, loved by the perfumer Maya Njie and the make-up artist Gucci Westman.

Experimental Perfume Club
experimentalperfumeclub.com
-
Release your inner scent alchemist and concoct your own perfume in Emmanuelle Moeglin's popular workshops.

Hermès
hermes.com
-
Refreshing colognes for all reasons and seasons from the ultimate artisanal brand.

Frédéric Malle
94 Greenwich Ave,
New York, NY 10011
fredericmalle.co.uk
-
The perfume 'publisher' works with renowned perfumers to create original scents as well as indulgent body oils, creams and candles. For the best experience, visit one of the stores, where you'll get an education in the power of smell.

Jo Malone London
jomalone.co.uk
-
Uplifting colognes that lend themselves to mix-and-match fragrance combining.

Maya Njie
mayanjie.com
-
Small-batch artisanal perfumes, inspired by the founder Maya Njie's Swedish and West African heritage.

Musée Lalique
40 rue du Hochberg,
67290 Wingen-sur-Moder
musee-lalique.com
-
A delightful museum for scent and design aficionados, with 250 Lalique perfume bottles on display.

Perfumer H
perfumerh.com
-
Lyn Harris's lovingly crafted natural perfumes and candles come in refillable (and engravable) hand-blown glass vessels.

Sana Jardin
sanajardin.com
-
This luxury fragrance company and women's cooperative uses a circular business model to empower its workforce by upcycling ingredient waste.

Santa Maria Novella
Via della Scala 16,
50123 Florence
buy.smnovella.eu
-
When in Florence, head to this centuries-old pharmacy for soaps, lotions and colognes.

Waft
waft.com
-
The online make-your-own-fragrance service using 'clean' practices and ingredients comes recommended by beauty writer Saleam Singleton.

Skincare and Body

79 Lux

79lux.com

-

*Founded by Karen Cummings-Palmer
to soothe her own skin problems,
79 Lux offers organic body oils and
balms formulated with wild ingredients.*

Aromatherapy Associates

aromatherapyassociates.com

-

*The best mood-boosting bath and shower
oils to reset or invigorate your mojo.*

Beauty Pie

beautypie.com

-

*Membership-based make-up and
skincare company selling innovative
formulations direct to the consumer at
great prices.*

Black Girl Sunscreen

blackgirlsunscreen.com

-

*An SPF30 sunscreen-moisturizer hybrid
formulated from natural ingredients for
people of colour, including children.*

Costa Brazil

livecostabrazil.com

-

*Skin-conditioning face and bodycare
products made from Brazil's hero oils,
nuts and resins.*

Margaret Dabbs

margaretdabbs.co.uk

-

*Considered podiatry royalty, Dabbs
also produces the best foot care products
in the business, including a bergamot-
infused foot scrub and the indestructible
professional foot file.*

Ecooking

ecooking.com

-

*Less-is-more Danish day creams, hand
creams and SPFs made from organic and
natural ingredients.*

Epara

eparaskincare.com

-

*Plagued by unidentified rashes, Epara's
founder, Ozohu Adoh, researched
African botanical ingredients – marula
oil from South Africa; moringa oil from
Kenya; argan oil from Morocco – to
produce her line of high-performance
skincare.*

Everyday Oil

everydayoil.com

-

*Multitasking oil for cleansing,
moisturizing and hair and beard
maintenance.*

Glow Recipe

glowrecipe.com

-

*This cruelty-free Korean-inspired
skincare uses antioxidant-rich fruit
extracts as the basis of its products. Try
the lightweight Watermelon Glow Pink
Juice Moisturizer for oil-free hydration.*

Dr Hauschka

drhauschka.co.uk

-

*No-nonsense therapeutic oils and rose
day creams are the consistent sellers of
this organic pharmacy brand.*

Hiki

hiki.com

-

*Inclusive bodycare and anti-perspirant
products co-created by its community.*

La Roche-Posay

laroche-posay.co.uk

-

*This drugstore favourite is famous for
its SPF and the gentle Toleriane line for
sensitive and allergy-prone skin.*

Liha

lihabeauty.com

-

*A British vegan beauty line with African
roots, the tuberose-infused Idan oil is the
multi-tasking hero item.*

Skincare and Body

Lush
lush.com

-

This fun beauty playground takes its consumption responsibilities seriously with packaging-light make-up, body- and skincare.

Omorovicza
omorovicza.co.uk

-

Beautifully restorative skincare harnessing the mineral-rich waters of Hungary. Try the mimosa-scented Miracle Facial Oil and Rejuvenating Night Cream.

REN
renskincare.com

-

The original 'clean' beauty brand (ren means 'clean' in Swedish), this bioactive skincare is increasingly sold in eco-conscious packaging.

Runako & Company
runakoandco.com

-

Body butters made from Zimbabwean beeswax, Ghanaian shea butter, organic cocoa butter and essential oils.

Shiro
shiro-shiro.uk

-

The Zen qualities of Shiro's stores are transported to your face and body in these beautifully formulated natural oils, powders and make-up balms.

Shiseido
shiseido.co.uk

-

One of the oldest cosmetics companies in the world, the Japanese brand is at the forefront of J-beauty skincare and make-up innovation.

Skin Gourmet
skingourmetgh.com

-

Raw, pure body butters, scrubs and oils from Accra.

Tata Harper
tataharperskincare.com

-

Boutique owner Linda V. Wright loves these effective yet kind-to-the-earth 'farm to face' skincare products.

The Inkey List
theinkeylist.com

-

Affordable and targeted skincare made from simple, functional ingredients.

Typology
uk.typology.com

-

Ingredient-light skincare oils and serums made sustainably in France. The direct-to-consumer model passes the savings on to the customer.

Uma
umaoils.com

-

These small-batch Ayurvedic treatment oils are grown, blended and bottled in India and crafted into masks, lip balms and cleansers.

Votary
Votary.co.uk

-

High performance skincare using premium plant oils. I recommend the indulgent yet potent bath and body oils and the Super Seed Facial Oil.

Weleda
weleda.co.uk

-

Weleda's biodynamic skincare – including its cult Skin Food moisturizer – is created according to nature's rhythms and natural systems, ensuring that no pesticides come into contact with the ingredients.

Haircare

Abhati
abhatisuisse.com
-
Indo-Swiss hair, face and body products made from fair-trade oils, with a proportion of profits going to local farms and education programmes.

Chāmpo
champohaircare.com
-
Chāmpo's capsule haircare line celebrates Ayurvedic principles for hair that looks and feels better.

Crown Affair
crownaffair.com
-
What started as a Google doc for Dianna Cohen's hair-obsessed friends became a hairbrush and oil line celebrating mindful rituals.

Dizziak
dizziak.com
-
The inclusive hair line of beauty journo-turned-entrepreneur Loretta De Feo caters for all hair types using vegan, plant-based ingredients.

David Mallett
14 Rue Notre Dame des Victoires, 75002 Paris
david-mallett.com
-
Achieve undone French-girl* hair with David Mallett's magical scissors, serums and Paris salon (*even though he's Australian).

Pattern
patternbeauty.com
-
Affordable, healthy haircare for the 'curly and coily' community, founded by the actor Tracee Ellis Ross.

Beauty Stores

Aēsop
aesop.com
-
Don't leave without your Resurrection Aromatique Hand Wash and lots of skincare samples for your best guy friend.

Buly 1803
6 Rue Bonaparte, 75006 Paris
buly1803.com
-
Herbal beauty oils and cosmetics from Ramdane Touhami and Victoire de Taillac-Touhami.

Content
32–4 New Cavendish Street, London W1G 8UE
contentbeautywellbeing.com
-
The ultimate workshop space and discovery destination for eco-conscious skintellectuals.

Dover Street Parfums Market
11 bis rue Elzévir, 75003 Paris
doverstreetparfumsmarket.com
-
Expect an unexpected clash of make-up, eco wellness, hi-tech skincare and mini exhibitions in this dedicated beauty playground.

Glossier
glossier.com
-
Part store, part hangout, Glossier's beauty boutiques are a destination for the 'no make-up make-up' crowd.

Lifestyle Stores

& Other Stories
256–8 Regent Street,
London W1B 3AF
stories.com
-
Stock up on bodycare, minimalist make-up and affordable perfumes from this Swedish high-street mecca.

Agnès B.
1 bis rue de Chaillot, 75016 Paris
agnesb.eu
-
Browse the signature stripy tees, jersey cardigans and art posters, then visit the nearby art foundation to view Agnès's famous contemporary art collection.

The Conran Shop
55 Marylebone High Street,
London W1U 5HS
conranshop.co.uk
-
All your bathroom needs are met here, from capacious towels to brushes, perfumes and handmade soaps.

Dover Street Market
18–22 Haymarket,
London SW1Y 4DG
(entrance on Orange Street)
london.doverstreetmarket.com
-
A happy collision of high fashion, street culture, niche perfumery and an artisan bakery, plus the best people-watching in town.

Japan House London
101-111 Kensington High Street,
London W8 5SA
japanhouselondon.uk
-
Immerse yourself in all things artisanal Japanese, from organic soaps and handmade brushes to fragrant teas.

Liberty
Regent Street,
London W1B 5AH
libertylondon.com
-
Lose yourself for hours in the beauty halls as you discover niche skincare and cult perfumes from Le Labo, Byredo and Nasomatto, among others.

Manufactum
manufactum.co.uk
-
Lose hours browsing German-crafted knick-knacks and no-nonsense bathroom kit designed to last a lifetime.

Merci
111 boulevard Beaumarchais,
75003 Paris
merci-merci.com
-
Pick up eco cleansers and browse the obscure fashion finds, then stay for a herbal tea overlooking the cobbled courtyard.

Mouki Mou
29 Chiltern Street,
London W1U 7PL
moukimou.com
-
A beautifully curated fashion, beauty and wellness boutique in London's villagey Chiltern Street.

Muji
muji.co.uk
-
The one-stop shop for all things bathroom storage and fuss-free J-Beauty skincare.

Native & Co.
116 Kensington Park Road,
London W11 2PW
nativeandco.com
-
De-stress the senses as you pick up handcrafted tea ceramics and bathroom accessories in this Japanese lifestyle destination.

Tiina The Store
tiinathestore.com
-
A masterclass in feel-good retail, selling everything from Perfumer H perfumes, Susanne Kaufmann's bath potions and vintage Marimekko quilts.

Make-up

Bobbi Brown
bobbibrown.co.uk
-
The original champion of 'no make-up make-up'. Stock up on the Extra Lip Tint balm sticks and the bestselling Skin Foundation Stick.

Chanel
chanel.com
-
Make-up minimalists, head for the Boy de Chanel products of no-nonsense basics for barely there (but beautiful) grooming.

Estée Lauder
esteelauder.co.uk
-
For long-lasting foundation in over 50 shades and the celebrated Advanced Night Repair serum, Estée Lauder still holds its own against younger start-ups.

Kure Bazaar
kurebazaar.com
-
High-shine, quick-drying nail colours formulated from wood pulp, wheat, corn, potatoes and cotton for those on a natural tip.

La Bouche Rouge
laboucherougeparis.com
-
The destination for perfect red lipsticks, all free from microplastics and designed to be refillable.

MAKE
makebeauty.com
-
Presenting skincare and cosmetics in a cultural context with future-thinking ingredients and formulations. Try the Dew Pots and Succulent Skin Gel.

NARS
narscosmetics.com
-
An inclusive range of foundations, concealers, blushers and lip colours in impeccable textures, for every skin tone.

Shakeup
shakeupcosmetics.com
-
Vegan make-up-meets-skincare for men.

Westman Atelier
westman-atelier.com
-
Gucci Westman's line of high-performance, ingredient-light make-up has skincare benefits to correct, heal and soothe.

Online Resources

The Beauty Conversation
instagram.com/thebeautyconversation
-
Industry insights and trend analysis from a positive community of beauty insiders.

Black Skin Directory
blackskindirectory.com
-
A trusted online resource connecting people of colour with reliable skincare professionals.

Idea Books
ideanow.online
-
The ultimate online inspiration destination for hard-to-get fashion, art and beauty books.

Inci Decoder
incidecoder.com
-
This ingredient-decoding directory is genius for deciphering your beauty product labels.

Into The Gloss
intothegloss.com
-
The original 'what's in my bathroom cabinet' source for curious skintellectuals.

Thingtesting
thingtesting.com
-
A fun discovery platform showcasing innovative direct-to-consumer start-ups from former venture capitalist Jenny Gyllander.

First published in Great Britain in 2021
by Laurence King Publishing
an imprint of The Orion Publishing Group Ltd
Carmelite House, 50 Victoria Embankment
London EC4Y 0DZ

An Hachette UK Company

13 5 7 9 10 8 6 4 2

© Text 2021 Navaz Batliwalla

© Illustrations 2021 Shira Barzilay

The moral right of Navaz Batliwalla to be identified as
the author of this work has been asserted in accordance
with the Copyright, Designs and Patents Act of 1988.

A CIP catalogue record for this book is
available from the British Library.

ISBN 978 1 91394 709 5

Design by Therese Vandling
Printed in China by C&C Offset Printing Co., Ltd.

Laurence King Publishing is committed to
ethical and sustainable production. We are
proud participants in The Book Chain Project®
bookchainproject.com

www.laurenceking.com
www.orionbooks.co.uk

Picture credits

All photography on pages 16–21, 58–61, 92–95 © Aria Isadora.
All photography on pages 22–25, 28–35, 98–103 © Robert
Rieger. All photography on pages 40–45, 112–117, 118–123
© Kasia Bobula. All photography on pages 48–53 © Alexander
Meininger. All photography on pages 64–69, 80–87 © Alfredo
Piola. All photography on pages 74–77 © Joseph Abbey-Mensah. All
photography on pages 108–111 © Demian Jacob.

Page 9 top left Todd Webb Archive; page 9 right 'Thoughtful Frida',
Hulton Archive via Getty images; page 9 bottom left *Nude Maria
Combing her Hair*, image courtesy of the artist, Francois Ghebaly
Gallery (Los Angeles) and Goodman Gallery (Johannesburg, Cape
Town and London); page 10 top left Amsterdam, Netherlands –
1976, Patti Smith, Gijsbert Hanekroot/Alamy Stock Photo; page 10
right Jean Michel Basquiat, 1985, © Roxanne Lowit; page 10 middle
left © Sukita; page 10 bottom *Jarvis* by Elizabeth Peyton at the
National Portrait Gallery, London, UK, Icona/Alamy Stock Photo;
page 12 Alternative Views – Milan Fashion Week Spring/Summer,
Vittorio Zunino Celotto/Getty; page 13 Torkil Gudnason; page 26
Josh Olins; page 46 Brigitte Lacombe; page 47 Frédéric Malle;
page 62 Aimee Shirley; page 78 © Brigitte Lacombe; page 96 Alexi
Lubomirski; page 97 Cire Trudon; page 124 Ellen von Unwerth,
photograph by Steffen Kugler.

Acknowledgements

I must first say a huge thank you to all the ritualists, their publicists
and managers for granting me access to their personal sanctuaries
and self-care secrets. Writing the bulk of this book during the 2020
pandemic was a challenge nobody could have foreseen and I'm
grateful for the support of everyone involved to steer it through to the
finish line. Thank you to Camilla Morton, Jo Lightfoot, Elen Jones,
Charlotte Selby and all at Laurence King and Orion Publishing for
the fantastic editing and publishing support. For design and picture
research, I bow down to Therese Vandling and Tory Turk. And for the
incredible photography that gives this book its rich intimacy, it was
an honour to work with Kasia Bobula, Robert Rieger, Alfredo Piola,
Demian Jacob, Alexander Meininger, Joseph Abbey-Mensah and Aria
Isadora. A heartfelt thank you goes to Shira Barzilay for the beautiful
illustrations throughout. For endless encouragement, brainstorming
sessions and expert advice there are too many people to name but a
special thanks to Shinobu Abe, Karen Cummings-Palmer, Charlotte
Ferguson, Shanu Walpita, Millie Kotseva, Teresa Havvas, Alison
Bishop, Yolanda O'Leary, Victoria Buchanan, Katie Service, David M
Watts and David Hill.

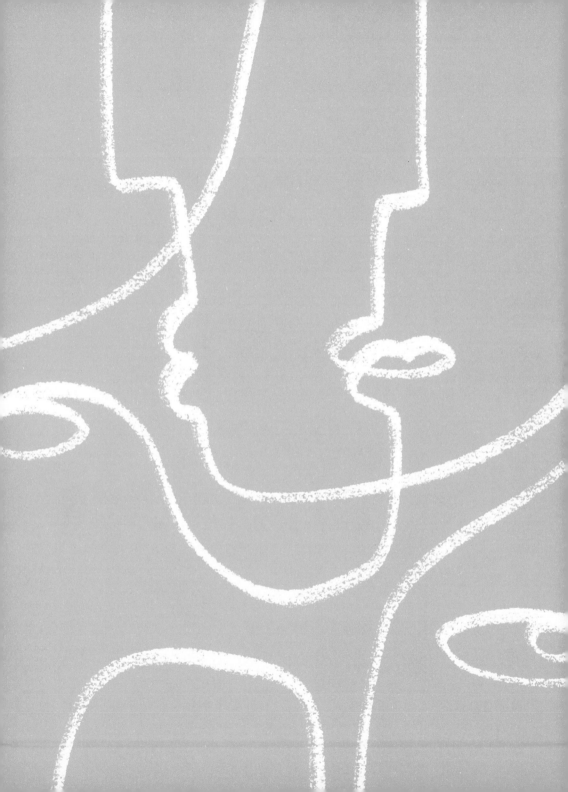

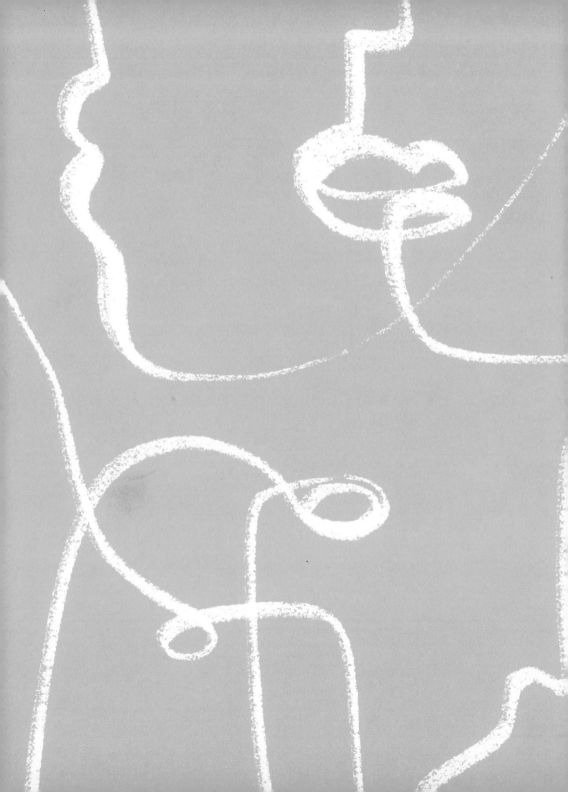